About the Authors

JOAN SAUERS The author of six nonfiction books about relationships, lifestyle, and wordplay, Joan suffered twenty years of chronic back pain until she finally found the right formula to maintain back health. She has also worked in Hollywood as a script reader and editor for Fox Studios and Zoetrope Studios, has run a production company in New York, and currently writes television and film screenplays. She also lectures at film schools in London, Paris, and Berlin in screenwriting. Born in New York, Joan lives in Sydney, Australia, with her daughter Ruby.

PETER EDWARDS, DO Born in Liverpool, England, Peter studied at the British School of Osteopathy in London before moving to Australia in 1991. Since 1998 he has been a lecturer in osteopathy at the University of Western Sydney and continues to work in private practice. An active sports-man, Peter spends most weekends doing yoga, kayaking, rock climbing, cycling, and racing up and down the coast (within the speed limit, of course) on his motorcycle.

Quick Fixes *for* EVERYDAY BACK PAIN

TIPS, TRICKS AND TREATMENTS TO STOP THE PAIN

JOAN SAUERS
with Peter Edwards, DO

MARLOWE & COMPANY
NEW YORK

QUICK FIXES FOR EVERYDAY BACK PAIN:
Tips, Tricks and Treatments to Stop the Pain

AVALON
publishing group incorporated

Contents

Muscle relaxants
Alcohol
Other drugs

Stop and rest
Move
Heat and cold
Massage
Relax
Medicate
Stretch/exercise
Listen

Posture
Stress management
Stretching
Basic back exercises
Inversion devices
Yoga
Tai chi and chi gung
Pilates
Alexander Technique
Feldenkrais
Walking
Running
Swimming and aquaerobics
Weight training
Other sports
Post-workout stretch
Magnesium and calcium

The biggest problem in the world could have been solved easily when it was small.

—Lao-Tzu

Introduction

*W*hy **another back** book? Because between 80 and 90 percent of us will experience back pain at least once in our lives. Because back trouble is most common among people of working age, between thirty-five and fifty-five. Because more and more children are affected by back problems. Because despite advances in diagnostic techniques, treatment, and preventative regimens, things are not getting better. And because we have yet to find a book on back care that the average non-doctor can understand and that includes an overview of different solutions to that universal problem: back pain.

Most back books are written from the point of view of the practitioners—doctors or physiotherapists or exercise gurus who have been successful with their techniques and want to share them with a wider audience. And while they all have things going for them, they do not necessarily give you the big picture—an overview of the variety of choices.

In addition to the experts, you'll have countless well-meaning friends, relatives, neighbors, and total strangers eager to tell you what they did about their back pain. It's good to listen because you may have some things in common. But ultimately, finding a solution is your responsibility because it's your back pain, and you are unique.

That's why we're not trying to sell you any single solution. We've seen different therapies work for some people and not others. In other words, we don't believe there's any one right way of doing things. This is certainly true of fixing your back. So, we're going to give you that overview and you can decide for yourself. We'll explain what the many practitioners who treat backs do, and tell you how they diagnose your problems. But don't worry. We won't get too technical. Just technical enough. Soon you can dazzle your friends with your knowledge of the difference between an osteopath and a chiropractor. Scoliosis and lordosis. Your glutes and your lats.

We'll also describe the many things you can do for yourself when back pain strikes. Arnica plasters, meditation, and a good old hot water bottle will soon be part of your antipain arsenal.

And last but not least, we'll let you in on all the fun things you can do to keep your pain from coming back, like yoga, walking, stretching, weights, tai chi, as well as exciting things with balls and cushions. In user-friendly, down-to-earth language with idiot-proof illustrations, this book should help you find a combination of solutions and preventative measures that's just right for you, so you can kiss your pain good-bye.

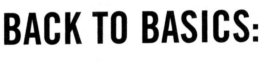

BACK TO BASICS:
What Is the Back?

$\mathcal{T}$ry to think holistically: this just means
seeing yourself as a whole rather than as
individual parts. Imagine that you're a mini-ecosystem of
mind, body, and spirit where everything is interconnected
and interdependent. The key to maintaining your little eco-
system is balance. Getting the balance right is the art of good
health. If there's an imbalance, the result can be back pain
or other health problems, from heart trouble to acne to
depression.

When we talk about "the back," we're referring to many
elements that work together, including the spine and other
bones, as well as muscles, ligaments, blood, and lymphatic
vessels, and other soft tissues from the neck to the bottom.
It's an incredibly intricate and complex system that has a
number of serious jobs to do.

Your back is your central stabilizer. It supports your head,
arms, and rib cage, and keeps your torso steady—and your
legs are attached at the bottom so it affects them too, and
they affect it. Your back resists force, carries weight, and

fights gravity. It can bend, twist, extend, and compress. No wonder, when you have a bad back, you're pretty useless. Everything depends on it. But for most of us, most of the time, in spite of its daunting responsibilities, the back does an amazing job. And most of that job is done by the spine.

THE SPINE

THINK OF THE spine as being the centerpiece of the body—literally and figuratively. It's situated in your center, and everything else hinges on it. It's strong but flexible, and more like a chain than a rod.

Attached to the skull at the top and the pelvis at the bottom, the spine is a column of small bones that houses the spinal cord, including its outer coverings (**meninges**) and outgoing nerve roots. The small bones are called **vertebrae**, and although they run continuously, we describe them in five different sections. From the top down, there are seven **cervical vertebrae** in the neck, twelve **thoracic vertebrae** in the upper and mid back, and five **lumbar vertebrae** in the lower back. It's useful to know these words because, when you go for treatment, they'll throw them around like you went to medical school. Below, in the pelvis, there are more vertebrae fused together in an area called the **sacrum**, and below that, more fused vertebrae in the **coccyx** or **tailbone**. The sacrum is a vital part of the pelvic girdle because it's the link between the lumbar spine and the legs.

Vertebrae all have a cylindrical part called the body, with flat upper and lower surfaces called **end plates**. Behind that is an arch with a ridgelike extension called the **spinous process**. These are the bony bumps down the center of your back that you can feel when you bend forward. On either side of the spinous process are the **facet joints**, which interlock and guide the vertebrae to keep them aligned.

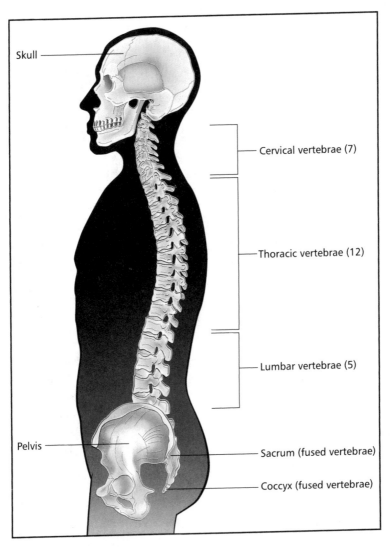

Skull

Cervical vertebrae (7)

Thoracic vertebrae (12)

Lumbar vertebrae (5)

Pelvis

Sacrum (fused vertebrae)

Coccyx (fused vertebrae)

Cervical or neck vertebrae are small and delicate to allow the head to turn (ideally!) in a 180-degree arc and support the head, while thoracic or upper and mid-back vertebrae are slightly larger. Your ribs are attached to these thoracic vertebrae, so that area of the back has the job of keeping the rib cage stable, which protects the heart, lungs, and other useful organs. The vertebrae of the lumbar zone, or lower back, are bigger and chunkier because they have to take the weight of the head, neck, arms, and torso as well as anything we carry, and also transfer that weight to the pelvis and legs. In addition, most of our bending is done from the lumbar region, so you can imagine why it's often the place where problems occur.

Between each pair of vertebrae, fused at the top and bottom, is a spongy pad called a **disc**. Discs keep vertebrae apart so they can move independently of each other. They also help control the vertebrae's range of movement, and absorb pressure when we're upright and even more when we lift or carry.

The disc has a jellylike center called the **nucleus pulposus**, which is encircled in a sheath called the **annulus fibrosus**. This sheath is a weave of fibers made mostly of collagen, and each fiber is stronger than a steel wire the same size. This is one reason discs are amazingly good at withstanding twists and compression. In fact, under extreme load (like when you try to lift your refrigerator when you're moving into your new house, or something equally clever) you're more likely to break your vertebral end plates before the annulus cracks.

And then there's the gooey nucleus of the disc. It's made of molecules that constantly try to suck in water and swell, but their capacity is limited by the pressure produced from the weight of your own body. So at night, when you're asleep and lying flat, there's nothing to curtail the absorption/swelling process. That's why in the morning you're always taller—your discs have expanded! It's also why astronauts can "grow" a few inches after a few days of weightlessness.

As we age, the soft center of the disc goes through some chemical changes, becoming at first mushy, then stringy, then solid.

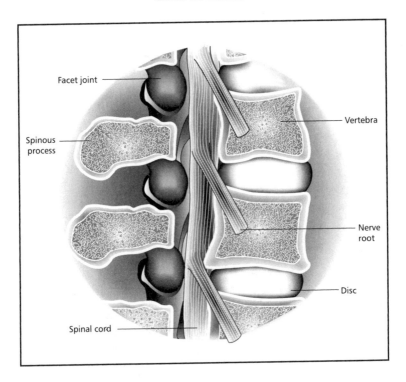

Facet joint

Spinous
process

Vertebra

Nerve
root

Disc

Spinal cord

Another hugely important function of the spine is to house and protect the spinal cord and nerve roots. Behind the vertebral bodies, in front of the vertebral arch, runs a hollow canal that contains the spinal cord. The spinal cord runs from the brain at the base of the skull through the spinal canal to the top of the second lumbar vertebra. Nerve bundles branch from the spinal cord between the vertebrae and extend to the rest of the body.

In healthy spines, both the spinal cord and nerves are sheathed in protective membranes that are crucial to proper functioning because the cord and nerves are responsible for carrying messages back and forth between the brain and every other tissue in the body. (It isn't hard to see why the back has to be looked at within the context of the whole body!)

LIGAMENTS, MUSCLES, AND FASCIA

FUNDAMENTAL TO THE complex network of structures known as the back are ligaments, muscles, and fascia. They play a huge part in keeping us upright, controlling movement, and absorbing load, and yet the role of these soft tissues is often underestimated, or even ignored, when defining what the back is.

As you've seen, the spine is an amazing piece of engineering but, without the dynamic collaboration of muscles and ligaments, it's like a marionette without strings—a sad, messy toppled pile of bones. Muscles and ligaments are the strings that empower our bones to move.

Ligaments are fibrous elastic bands of tissue that link vertebrae to each other and help stabilize the spine. In partnership, an intricate system of muscles initiates and directs movement, bears weight, and helps to keep the spine in proper alignment. Like ligaments, **muscles** are also fibrous bands, but they are even more flexible. Each of us has an amazing weave of muscles, including small ones that lie very deep and extend from the spine, such as the multifidus muscles, to larger outer muscles, like the latissimus dorsi.

Some of the most important muscles of the back and associated structures that you might be familiar with, include:

- the "lats" (**latissimus dorsi**), which extend from the upper back to the lumbar region along the outer sides of the back
- the "glutes" (**gluteus maximus**), a.k.a. muscles in your buttocks
- **deltoids,** which cover the outer shoulders
- **trapezius muscles,** which run along the tops of your shoulders, and from your shoulders inward toward the spine

- **rhomboids,** which run from the spine to the border of each shoulder blade
- **erector spinae,** which are deep muscles that run parallel to the spine and hold it erect
- **piriformis,** an important muscle that connects the sacrum to the hip and is often involved with sciatic nerve problems
- **neck extensors,** those vertical muscles at the back of the neck that can feel like titanium bands after a long day at the computer
- **neck flexors,** which extend down the side of the neck toward the front
- **hamstrings,** which are the big muscles in the backs of our thighs

Although they're not part of the back, it's impossible not to include the abdominal muscles and the diaphragm in any discussion about backs, because their role in maintaining healthy back function is so critical. Some practitioners call the abdominals and diaphragm our "second back" or our "front back," because when they're strong and toned they do the same job as the back muscles—directing movement, bearing weight, and keeping everything nicely aligned.

To do all this, abdominal muscles spread vertically and diagonally across the stomach in crisscrossing diagonal lines. In collaboration, the diaphragm is a domelike sheath of muscles and tendons connected to your lower ribs and upper lumbar spine. Together, they do an amazing job.

If you place your fingers gently somewhere along your lumbar spine and contract your abdominal muscles, you can feel the spine being supported from the front. If you do this while taking or holding a deep breath, like weightlifters do, you can really feel the support. What you're doing is using your abdominals, diaphragm, and lungs like an internal air bag to cushion and support the spine. Contraction of the abdominals also lifts the spine vertically, to prevent too much compression. So when we talk about the back and the muscles involved in its function, we can't forget the "abs."

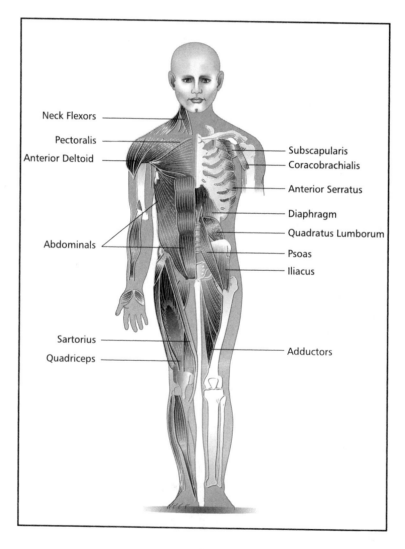

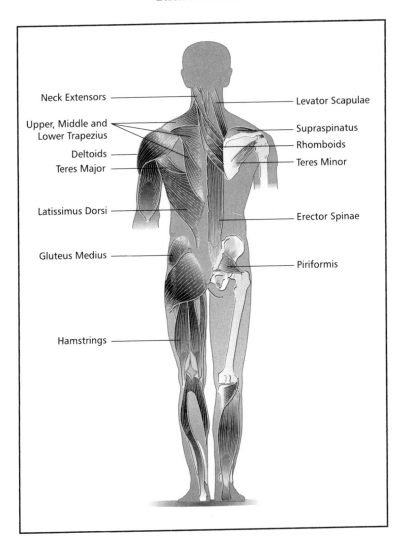

Neck Extensors

Upper, Middle and
Lower Trapezius

Deltoids

Teres Major

Latissimus Dorsi

Gluteus Medius

Hamstrings

Levator Scapulae

Supraspinatus

Rhomboids

Teres Minor

Erector Spinae

Piriformis

Fascia is the extensive network of fibroelastic tissue that connects, separates, and contains all bones, organs, and other tissues of the body. It serves to enhance the function of the muscles and joints, maintaining posture and coordinating smooth movement.

When the spine is in good working order with the help of muscles, ligaments, and fascia, it forms a sort of stretched-out S-shape, and is quite beautifully designed to perform its many extraordinary jobs. But of course life isn't always simple or easy to manage, and our back sometimes isn't in good working order. So as much fun as you're having with all this technical jargon (wasn't too difficult, was it?), it's time we moved on to the real reason for this book: your pain!

2 BACK PAIN:
Kinds and Causes

*I*t's not surprising that most of us have bad backs at some point in our lives, and we can blame evolution for that. It's only relatively recently that human beings started to live past twenty-five or thirty years of age. If we still died young, most of us would never have back pain, as it often doesn't occur until after the age of around thirty-five. Fortunately, most of us don't die young anymore. Advances in lifestyle, nutrition, medicine, and really warm pajamas have brought us to an average lifespan in the U.S. of seventy-seven! And remember that we're the only species to walk upright (most of the time). Walking and doing all the other stuff we do upright—like carrying heavy loads, working on assembly lines, and sitting at computers over a period of *decades*—is bound to lead to spinal compression and back trouble. It's just one of the by-products of living in the twenty-first century and not fifty thousand years ago.

WHAT IS BACK PAIN?

PAIN IS A signal that something is wrong with you. Sounds simple, doesn't it? Unfortunately, the causes of back pain usually aren't as simple as other kinds of pain, and you can probably understand why after reading the previous chapter. Being as complicated as it is, the back has a lot of different bits and pieces that can go haywire. Back pain isn't like a broken arm or a black eye or a cut knee. It isn't as easily visualized, isolated, diagnosed, or treated.

For those of you who haven't had the pleasure of giving birth, back pain is also often the worst pain you'll ever have. This is due to a combination of the kind of injury you have and the fact that we use our backs for everything, including lying down, sitting, standing, walking, and every tiny movement in between. Our backs even come into play when we're breathing, which it's nice to do fairly constantly.

And aside from the fact that it hurts like hell, back pain prevents you from having fun (break-dancing, snowboarding, and sex are usually off the menu when you have a bad back). It's also the second leading cause for absenteeism from work in the U.S.—head colds came in first.

Also, back pain comes in lots of shapes and sizes. It might be sharp, jagged, shocking, burning, deep, piercing, dull, throbbing, pinpoint, wide-ranging, brief, or endless. In short, back pain is incredibly individual, and only you know exactly what it feels like.

But don't despair!

The good news is that most back pain is not serious and in the huge majority of cases, it will either go away on its own or with minimal treatment. Often, the exact cause of your pain will remain a mystery. But if you experience back pain, it's probably a good idea to have some understanding of the variety of possible causes so you can deal with things in an educated way and avoid it in the future.

The following descriptions of various conditions are not meant to alarm you. Of course we're aware that, while knowledge is power, a little bit of knowledge can be a dangerous thing: we don't want you reading this and then deciding that you have some serious chronic spinal disease when all you have is a muscle spasm from painting the kids' bedroom all day. That's why it's important for you to understand how to use this information. In no way is it meant to replace the diagnosis or treatment of your practitioner. Instead, we want to empower you with enough understanding so that when problems do arise, you can cope with them better and work more closely with the health professional you're comfortable with. And next time, get the kids to help with the painting!

SOFT-TISSUE STRAIN

IT'S FAIRLY EASY to strain soft tissues of the back, such as ligaments, muscles, and tendons, and the symptoms are often referred to as "nonspecific back pain." Usually these episodes are short and often won't recur. Short episodes like this are described as "acute" back pain.

Although it's nothing to laugh about, this kind of strain isn't a tragedy and will either heal by itself or with basic treatment, as long as the activity or position that caused the strain is changed.

Strains like these can come from overuse, bad posture, or a sudden awkward movement like a fall. Gardening, tiling, painting, lifting heavy objects, and doing sport or exercise when you're out of shape are typical causes. Sometimes the pain will flare up a day or two after you've done the heavy work.

Being out of shape is probably the most common contributing factor. Weak back and abdominal muscles mean that, if you're lifting or carrying, the spine has to take the whole load. The spine is also unprotected if back and abdominal muscles are not able to control movement and stabilize your upper body. This is how ligaments can become overstretched or torn. They can be easily damaged by sudden or awkward movement—and unfortunately, ligaments will take longer to heal than muscles because their blood supply isn't as good. Also, they don't recoil back to their original length, but stay stretched out, allowing for less support and further strain.

This kind of injury usually starts with a sharp pain that eventually fades to a dull ache, with some incidental muscle spasms, swelling, and inflammation thrown in for good measure.

Or, your pain might come on gradually. This is often caused by habitual poor posture, like slumping at your computer and having an unsupported lower back. You might have felt stiffness before real pain set in, but you ignored it. Deadlines have to be met, right?

Pain that is persistent and lasts for a long time, at least several months, is called chronic pain and can seriously affect you and your lifestyle. There can be many causes, including the following conditions.

HYPERMOBILITY

YOU KNOW HOW there was always some show-off at school who could put her feet behind her head and everybody thought it was cool? Well, that person may today be paying the price for naturally loose limbs that can result in back pain.

When people are born with looser, more flexible ligaments than normal, it's called hypermobility. Because the ligaments don't hold the joints securely in place, the joints can move too far before the muscles are forced to stabilize them.

This can lead to joint strain and symptoms of repetitive irritation and inflammation. Also, those poor overworked muscles have to stay contracted and tight (also known as hypertonic) to make up for the lazy ligaments. This means that muscle spasm, soreness, and stiffness are very common in someone who is hypermobile, and they can also get very tired because their muscles are constantly being over-worked.

People like ballet dancers and gymnasts are often hyper-mobile, which is why they started doing what they do in the first place. Or their hypermobility can be a by-product of overtraining at an early age. The point is that sometimes they suffer the effects of their loose limbs as much as they do from injuries sustained doing all that bouncing, twirling, and leaping about. It's sort of a chicken-and-egg problem, and maybe not worth determining which came first. The important thing is how awful it feels when it hurts.

HERNIATED AND PROLAPSED DISCS

IF A DISC'S outer layer (the annulus) weakens, it can bulge out from in between two vertebrae when sufficient pressure is exerted. This is called a herniated disc, and can bring on some pretty nasty pain. If this condition progresses so that the annu-lus actually tears, allowing the center to ooze out, it's called a ruptured or prolapsed disc. This is what used to be called a "slipped disc," but most people don't use that description anymore because it's not accurate: discs don't slip.

It's hard to rupture a disc with a blow, but it can happen with repeated stress or pressure, also known as fatigue failure. This is particularly common if the repeated movement occurs with your back in a bent or twisted position. It's the same as with a piece of wire. If you bend or twist and straighten it once, it's fine; but if you do it over and over, the metal will eventually break easily. This is why a rupture can occur just by lifting a book or a glass of water: it's the straw that breaks the camel's back. And unfortunately, you're the camel.

Because there are no nerves inside a disc, the pain doesn't actually come from the disc itself. What happens is that normal compression of the spine forces the herniated disc to bulge, or the nucleus of the ruptured disc to squeeze out, so that it presses on a nerve root or the spinal cord. This is what hurts so much. And it can be especially tricky isolating the offending disc if a nerve is involved, because your pain might not be where the actual contact between disc and nerve is. Nerves are interwoven in complex patterns up and down the spine so that you may feel pain in one place, but the source is actually some place else. This is called referred pain—it starts somewhere other than where you feel it.

Pain from a herniated or prolapsed disc can be excruciating. Often it will start out as stiffness or soreness or even a muscle spasm and then suddenly there may be what feels like a little pop or explosion. If it occurs when you're bending over, you might feel stuck, unable to straighten up. It's a miserable condition.

Not only can you get intense pain, you can experience tingling and numbness in arms, hands, legs, and feet, and in the worst case, loss of bowel or bladder control, which is a serious medical emergency that requires surgery. Talk about adding insult to injury!

Usually, pain from a damaged disc will subside slowly, but because the annulus doesn't regenerate, there's always the danger that if extreme compression occurs again, you'll find yourself in agony. The peak age for disc trouble is between twenty-five and forty, and it plagues men more than women.

FIBROMYALGIA

WIDESPREAD PAIN IN the back, neck, and across the shoulders, which also often affects the hip, elbow, and knee joints, is called fibromyalgia. It can be associated with chronic fatigue and other symptoms such as irritable bowels, sleep disorders, depression, and migraine headaches. Although its cause hasn't been clearly identified, sufferers seem to have poor circulation, therefore too little oxygen in their muscle cells. They also break down muscle protein at a faster than normal rate, which could cause pain and fatigue. The condition may also relate to diet, allergies, a virus, and some evidence even blames dysfunctional sleep rhythms; however, that may be an effect rather than a cause.

REPAIR DAMAGE AND SCARRING

Bones

Sometimes, after a strain or injury, the natural repair process can go too far and change the back's structures, limiting the spine's range of movement. In these cases, pain comes from excessive bony growth around the affected joints rather than from the original injury. This excess can press on nerves and ligaments, causing inflammation and pain.

Ligaments and fascia (collagen)

When torn or damaged collagen fibers heal, scar tissue can form that is thicker and less flexible than the original fiber. This area is called an adhesion, and it can be painful or stiff when stretched.

Other soft tissue

In some disorders, the protective layers around the spinal cord or nerve roots can become inflamed and thickened with scar tissue. This condition has the lovely name, arachnoiditis, and it can cause major pain in the back, legs, and arms in similar fashion to meningitis.

Often soft-tissue scarring that follows abdominal surgery (for example, a bowel or hernia operation or caesarian), can lead to postural change that can cause back pain. Another reminder of how every part of us affects every other part!

WHIPLASH

THE MOST COMMON reason for whiplash is a car accident. A sudden impact forces the head to swing back and forth, yanking the neck with it, but the cervical muscles don't have time to engage. What usually result are strained ligaments and muscle spasms, but they'll normally fade within a few days or weeks, depending on the severity of the accident and other factors. Occasionally, whiplash can cause more serious injuries, such as disc or nerve damage, or even trauma to the spinal cord. Whiplash symptoms can often be delayed until hours or even days later when they can gradually worsen. In these cases treatment is necessary.

SCIATICA

ALTHOUGH THE LOWER neck can also have its fair share of disc problems, nerve roots at the bottom of the lumbar spine are the ones most often affected by pesky discs: the lower back takes most of our abuse in the way of lifting and bending. The base of the lumbar spine is where we find the roots that form the sciatic nerve, which runs down the leg. Sharp pain that runs from the lower back down the back of the leg is called sciatica, and a damaged disc is sometimes the culprit.

Although sciatica can be brought on by disc trouble, there are other causes. The thing to remember is that sciatica is not a disease, it's a symptom. Imbalance in the pelvis and hips, inflammation of the sacroiliac joints, spinal curvature, and spasms in the gluteals or piriformis muscles are all possible reasons that the sciatic nerve comes under pressure and results in that searing, grabbing pain in the lower back, buttocks, and/or legs.

SCOLIOSIS, LORDOSIS, AND KYPHOSIS

WE USE THREE different terms for spinal curvature: scoliosis, lordosis, and kyphosis, and they all have very different causes and effects. Within limits, curvature is normal, and won't cause problems. But beyond a certain point, radical twists and turns of the spine will result in pain and loss of function.

When the spine is curved to one side or another instead of straight when seen from behind, it's called scoliosis. Some people are born with it, or it could be brought on gradually by having one leg shorter than the other, or even by bad postural habits. With scoliosis there's usually a curve in the lower back, then a compensating curve in the opposite direction in the upper back. Some degree of scoliosis is so common that it's actually considered normal. But extreme cases will cause pain and require treatment.

Extreme pain from scoliosis occurs when the vertebrae get jammed up, facet joints become chronically inflamed, and ligaments and muscles are unevenly stressed. And we're not talking about just one spot. Because of the domino effect up and down the whole spine, people with scoliosis can have neck pain, headaches, shoulder and arm pain, pain up and down the back, and sciatica.

The other terrible thing about scoliosis is that it can strike children as young as nine or ten and get progressively worse if left untreated.

In contrast, lordosis and kyphosis are words to describe natural curvature, but as pathological conditions they also refer to extreme curvature that can often come on in adulthood and cause trouble. Lordosis describes too much lower inward curvature, and kyphosis is too much upper forward curvature. Pain from these conditions can come from compression, inflammation, and soft tissue strain, and can get worse if untreated. In later life, they can even lead to breathing difficulties, exhaustion, headaches, and a multitude of other health problems.

SPONDYLOSIS AND OSTEOARTHRITIS

SPONDYLOSIS IS A fancy word to describe the normal wear and tear that occurs within the spine over a lifetime, and while it may result in back pain, it also may not. So it's not a disease—unless ageing itself is a disease, and we are philosophically opposed to that point of view!

Over the years, the vertebral end plates develop a rim of bone around the edge of the disc, and the discs and facet joints deteriorate as well. They lose their lubrication and become rough, therefore not as efficient. This deterioration of the bones and soft tissue is called osteoarthritis.

Spondylosis and osteoarthritis usually occur together. These changes are most common in older people and in the lumbar or cervical spine because that's where most of the action has been over the decades. Because the bone mass around the discs and facet joints has built up, movement becomes restricted and stiffening can occur. Sciatica and other effects of disc damage might also result, and there can be some inflammation and injury of nearby soft tissue.

The weird thing is that some people whose tests reveal a lot of spondylosis and osteoarthritis might have no pain at all, whereas others who appear to have little evidence of the conditions can be in agony. It's a little like chaos theory. There are so many variables that can affect your back that it's often virtually impossible to determine exactly what series of events over a lifetime has led to your present state of pain.

FRACTURES

SOMETIMES A TRAUMATIC event can lead to fractures of bones in the spine. A bad fall, a car crash, or a direct hit to the back can be very bad news. We all know that joker who will pull the chair out from under someone as he or she is sitting down, resulting in a fall on the buttocks, possibly causing a disc herniation or fracture of the coccyx. This is often a very painful and inconvenient injury, especially when you want to do pretty ordinary things like sit down or move your bowels. You don't even want to think about it.

The strange thing is that sometimes there is terrible pain as a result of fractures to bones in the spine, and sometimes there is none. Obviously if the spinal cord or nerve roots are irreparably damaged there can be paralysis, but breaks to the bones themselves are usually not irreparable. Vertebral fractures due to osteoporosis occur often and are left alone to heal themselves. The aftereffects are usually a local reduction in movement and a greater tendency to slump.

Much more common than the traumatic break is a micro-fracture in a vertebral arch at the back of the spinal column, or in one of the vertebrae. This kind of break will often not even show up in X-rays; with rest and proper treatment, the bone will heal.

Sometimes, however, a break in the arch will destabilize a vertebra, which can then slide forward or back, pulling on ligaments and stretching nerve roots. This is a spondylolis-thesis. To make the understatement of the year, this doesn't feel very nice.

OSTEOPOROSIS

IF BONES BECOME porous, they become brittle and weak, and small breaks can take place when the bones are under even a small amount of pressure. This is called osteoporosis, and it's fairly widespread, especially among women after they go through menopause, usually after the age of fifty (although they can develop osteoporosis at a younger age). Men can have it too.

Because the spine is always under pressure (even when we're lying down, it's busy keeping us stable), our vertebrae are especially prone to fractures from osteoporosis. Vertebrae can actually be crushed by the weight of the body, but only when there is very little bone mass left. This can result in dreadful back pain, loss of height, and that stooped posture you sometimes see in older sufferers.

Osteoporosis can be caused by hormonal conditions, lack of exercise, disease, long-term steroid use, too much protein in the diet, and calcium deficiency. A recent Australian study showed that rural residents suffer up to one-third fewer fractures through osteoporosis than their urban counterparts, due to a combination of more exercise and greater exposure to sunlight. Sunlight increases our concentrations of vitamin D, which enhances muscle strength and helps our bones absorb calcium from the bloodstream. So, in our rush to stay out of the sun and avoid skin cancer, we might be shortchanging other aspects of our health.

SPINAL STENOSIS

SOME PEOPLE ARE born with or can develop an unusually narrow spinal canal, which makes it easier for nerve roots to be pressed by spinal structures. Other people can develop the condition as an accompaniment to their osteoarthritis. Either way, it can lead to back and limb pain along with numbness, tingling, and sciatica. And because increased blood flow can compress nerves even further, the pain can get worse during exercise and then better after resting.

Pain from spinal stenosis can worsen when arching backward, because in that position, the spinal canal gets smaller. That's why sufferers with this condition can feel better when they cycle rather than walk, as the canal gets slightly bigger when one is bent forward.

ANKYLOSING SPONDYLITIS

ANKYLOSING SPONDYLITIS IS often detected among younger people, typically men between around twenty and forty, although women can have it too. It's actually a form of arthritis, and causes inflammation as well as changes in the ligaments, usually starting in the joints between the sacrum and pelvis, then moving up the spine. It can lead to overall stiffening as well as a painful stoop. Often, pain caused by ankylosing spondylitis will be relieved by exercise. Also, it is a progressive disease, so it's important to keep up exercise and treatment that can slow or even stop it in its tracks.

HORMONES AND PREGNANCY

WOMEN OFTEN HAVE lower back pain just before their period is due because of increased levels of prostaglandins—hormones that have a range of effects such as swelling, cramping, and inflammation of the uterus. All of these can cause referred pain. Typically, it's in the lumbar and sacral region, especially the sacroiliac joints, where we often have these lovely monthly visitations of pain and swelling.

The effects of hormones on a woman's body and particularly her back become even more extreme during pregnancy, when ligaments become soft and loose. And then there's the extra weight of the growing baby, as well as added fluid in the breasts. All this increases compression on the vertebrae and discs, and puts greater strains on muscles, which are already coping with slack ligaments. So many, if not most, pregnant women will have to deal with some degree of back pain, which is why loving partners who are also enthusiastic massage therapists are in such great demand.

INFLEXIBILITY AND LACK OF FITNESS

IF BEARING WEIGHT is one of the things that causes spinal compression, and spinal compression can lead to various types of back pain, then it seems logical that too much body weight can contribute to a bad back. But funnily enough, studies have been inconclusive about the connection between obesity and back pain. What are clearly much greater contributors to back pain are inflexibility and lack of fitness, which can afflict thin people as well as heavy ones.

Being out of shape means that the back and abdominal muscles that are supposed to direct and control movement as well as stabilize upper body structures are not up to the job. Sadly, the result can be frequent soft tissue strain, and eventually more serious long-term back problems. Another surprise is that even more than strength, flexibility is the key to maintaining a healthy back. Without a supple back, good posture and a healthy range of movement are impossible. Bad posture and poor range of movement cause back pain.

STRESS

HERE IS WHERE thinking holistically will really help you understand back pain. In a lot of cases, the conditions that we've already talked about, like a huge range of soft-tissue strain, disc trouble, and even obesity, can be brought on by stress. And where other diseaselike conditions exist, stress will make them worse. Foolishly, we like to think of stress as something that lives in our head—that can be isolated and kept in some kind of escape-proof box. But it can't. It leaks out to the rest of our body.

Stress can lead to heart disease, stomach and bowel disorders, and be a major contributing factor in a variety of cancers. Unmanaged stress certainly lowers our immune systems.

NASA scientists recently concluded that stress and psycho-emotional issues contribute to 98 percent of all diseases.

One of the most common ways in which people deal with their stress is by tensing muscles. With some people, this tension concentrates in the neck and shoulders. For others, it might be right between their shoulder blades. And for others, all their anxiety is focused in the small of their backs.

All this muscle tension will lead to back pain if it's not dealt with. And then it's a vicious cycle of stress leading to pain, which in turn leads to more stress, which then yields more pain.

SMOKING

THERE ARE SEVERAL recent studies that make a connection between smoking and bad backs, and it's just one more nail in the coffin for the tobacco lobbies. Smoking reduces blood flow around the discs so that they lose their bounciness and prematurely age. Reduction of blood flow also means that your muscles are getting fewer nutrients and less oxygen, which means that they're less efficient. Smoking inhibits healing and causes muscle fatigue. Another factor is coughing, which strains the soft tissues and can even pull structures out of alignment . . . So if the threats of cancer, heart disease, and wrinkles aren't enough to scare you off cigarettes, maybe the specter of back pain is.

OTHER CONDITIONS

ONCE AGAIN, BECAUSE the back has so many different components with different functions, and those components are connected to so many other sites in our bodies, there are still dozens more reasons you can get back pain.

Neural Compression syndrome describes the sensation of tingling, pins and needles in the arms and legs that can be associated with a bad back.

You might have a bacterial infection in the spinal cord, which can cause osteomyelitis—a disease with flulike symptoms.

Pneumonia and other bronchial conditions can lead to back pain, as can mastitis, an inflammation of the mammary gland.

Or there's rheumatoid arthritis—a persistent inflammation of the joints.

Although relatively rare, tumors can also produce severe back pain.

Diabetes, which affects the pancreas, can lead to back trouble where that organ's nerves are rooted in the spinal cord, and a similar phenomenon can occur with stomach ulcers and a variety of uterine complaints.

Most common among older people, Paget's disease accelerates bone growth causing it to press on nerve roots and ligaments, resulting in pain. And if that weren't bad enough, the new bone is softer than normal growth, so it can break easily, especially in the spine.

And then there's simple gravity. It's a sad fact for tall people that they have more back pain than short people.

Back pain may result as a combination of a couple or more conditions we've mentioned, which on their own might not create problems. There are other things that can contribute to back pain, but we've got to draw the line somewhere. We want to educate, not inundate. Ultimately, especially with pain that doesn't go away after a few days or is accompanied by other serious symptoms, you need to consult a health practitioner about your back. At least now you'll have some idea of what they're talking about, and of course it's never a bad idea to let them know you've done a little reading yourself.

3 HOW TO STOP THE PAIN

$\mathcal{W}$hile their back pain may be distinctly different, all sufferers have one thing in common: they want it to stop! Whether it's from a traumatic injury, a herniated disc, or osteoporosis, back pain is something that no one likes and no one should have to put up with. Luckily, in most cases, back pain can be eliminated. Depending on your condition and its severity, it may take some dedication and often a willingness to try different therapies and collaborate with a practitioner or two to become pain-free. But you can do it. Pain is a great motivator.

There's a lot that you can do yourself to relieve your own pain, which we'll get to a little later. But if you haven't experienced serious back pain before and it's not going away after a day or two, or if it's nothing new but your usual methods for relief aren't working, it's best to consult a professional. Also, you should get in to see a practitioner soon if you have sciatica, or swelling and pain in parts of your body in addition to your back. Sometimes it's hard to get an appointment when you want one, but there are certain symptoms that demand immediate medical attention, and if you can't get in to see someone right away, you can always go to the emergency room of your local hospital. If you have any of the following symptoms, get in your car now:

- ◆ Your pain is the result of a fall, an accident (e.g., a car or industrial mishap), or other sudden impact injury.
- ◆ You felt severe pain after lifting something heavy.
- ◆ You have back pain, plus decreased muscle function in your legs or feet.
- ◆ You have back pain, plus numbness or tingling in the lower half of your body.
- ◆ You have back pain that keeps you up at night but goes away when you exercise, plus fever and chills.
- ◆ You have altered bowel or bladder control.

In the following section, we'll describe some of the different techniques that various practitioners use to relieve your pain and set you on the road to recovery. As we said earlier, we believe each discipline has something to offer. It's the individual skill and insight of the practitioner as much as the discipline or philosophy he or she chooses to follow that really seem to make the most difference. There are great osteopaths and ordinary osteopaths. Great orthopedic surgeons and ordinary ones. Just like singers or dancers or car mechanics. This is why it's always a good idea to ask around when you're in the market for a back pain specialist. And don't worry. There will be no shortage of people who will love sharing their experiences with you. If the same name keeps popping up when people rave about some miracle-worker, make an appointment.

The other factors of course are your own personal beliefs and preferences. For some, gentle manipulation is their favored back therapy. Others like the traditional Chinese approach with herbal medicine and acupuncture. Still others feel most comfortable with more conventional Western techniques including anti-inflammatory medication and traction. The good news is that they can all get results. And always remember that the goal of treatment should be to become independent of that treatment.

Our goal is to give you enough information so that you can decide what treatment will best suit you. There's a lot of interdisciplinary rivalry and suspicion out there, and practitioners sometimes dismiss each other's techniques or philosophies as either total or partial garbage. The thing to remember is that it's your responsibility to educate yourself as best you can. Then you can be the judge, based on results.

We also want to make things easier once you're in the practitioner's office. The more you know, the better equipped you'll be to describe your pain and help them understand your condition. The more they know, the better equipped they'll be to aid your recovery.

HOW TO MAKE THE MOST OUT OF YOUR VISIT TO A PROFESSIONAL

THE FIRST IMPORTANT thing to do before rushing off to any back-care professional is to get your head in the right place. We're not talking about where it sits on your spine, we're talking about attitude. Research shows that people who take responsibility for their back care and see their relationship with practitioners as a collaboration get the best results. There isn't a surgeon or physiotherapist or chiropractor or other therapist alive who can cure you without your help.

So increase your chance of a full recovery by helping the practitioner do his or her job.

Before your visit
◆ Gather any medical records that might be relevant including X-rays (even old ones), blood tests, scans, etc.

◆ Write a list of your symptoms as well as the approximate dates they appeared, including any loss of function.
◆ Write a short description of your medical history including all the big events, even if they don't seem connected to your current complaint.
◆ Write a list of any medications, herbs, vitamins, or minerals you're taking.
◆ Write down any questions you have.
◆ Dress in clothes and shoes that are easy to take off. You may need to change into a gown for an examination, and you don't want to make your injury worse by fiddling with buttons at your back, or bending over to unlace knee-high boots.

The reason for writing all that stuff down is that it's so easy to forget a small detail that may have enormous significance to your practitioner. An old fall off a bicycle, tingling in your toes, a lack of magnesium in your diet—any of these things might help an expert diagnose your problem and come up with a solution. And if you forget one of these things during your visit, you're not likely to call later and say, "Oh yeah, and there was also that time on my twenty-first birthday when I took a flying leap off a . . ." So make lists.

During your visit

◆ Refer to your lists, and be completely honest. Embarrassing things like incontinence or pain during sex are critical details in your back picture, and—trust us—practitioners have heard it all before.
◆ Stick to the point. You might enjoy showing pictures of your kids, but if you've done your lists properly, you'll need every minute of the visit to explore your case.
◆ Write down the practitioner's advice so you don't forget something important later like those fun abdominal

exercises or the fact that you should only take anti-inflammatories with food.

◆ Ask questions. Not just the ones on your list, but any that spring to mind during the visit when your practitioner starts talking about your "contracting ligamentum flavum."

Follow these handy hints and you'll be a more empowered patient. Otherwise, you're wasting your money and their time.

GENERAL PRACTICE

IF YOU'VE NEVER had back pain before now, your first stop might be your general practitioner. A GP will ask you questions about your pain and any other symptoms or associated conditions, and how the pain came on. In the large majority of cases, he or she won't call for an X-ray. If your pain is "non-specific," not too severe, and there is no history of back trouble, he or she might just tell you to rest, apply ice or heat (depending on how long ago the pain started and what caused it), take some painkillers or anti-inflammatory medication, and follow up with some gentle stretching and other exercise. Most medications GPs would recommend are available over the counter, but obviously they'll write a prescription if they think you need something stronger.

Or, your GP might refer you to someone else like a physiotherapist or possibly a complementary practitioner such as an osteopath or chiropractor. More and more GPs are referring patients to acupuncturists, and some GPs actually practice acupuncture as part of the treatment they offer.

If your condition is more serious or demands immediate specialist assessment, your GP might refer you to an orthopedic surgeon.

In some cases, your GP might recognize stress, depression,

or another psychological condition as a contributing factor in your back pain. In this case, referrals and recommendations are in order.

A huge and fairly recent leap forward is that an increasing number of GPs suggest some form of meditation, as they recognize that stress is a common contributing factor in back pain. This is very smart advice that could change your life and your general health for the better.

OSTEOPATHY

BORN IN 1828 in Virginia, Andrew Taylor Still was a doctor who recognized that traditional medicine wasn't working in an unacceptably high percentage of cases. He was particularly horrified by the practice of administering monstrous dosages of crude drugs for all sorts of ailments that he believed they didn't cure. He tried a lot of different techniques and eventually developed a form of physical treatment for which he coined the term "osteopathy." In 1892, he founded the first osteopathic school.

Osteopathy is now a widely accepted, highly effective holistic system of diagnosis and treatment for pain sufferers. In fact, although they can treat a wide variety of health problems from bronchitis to gynecological or visceral disorders, back pain is the most common reason that people visit osteopaths. If you have trouble involving muscles, joints, ligaments, tendons, adhesions, nerves, circulation, or inflammation, you will be in good hands with an osteopath.

In the U.S., osteopaths are fully certified physicians and are licensed to perform surgery and prescribe medicine, but they're also trained in manipulation of the musculoskeletal system. In Australia and Great Britain, osteopaths are not medical doctors but are more thoroughly trained in what is called "ten-fingered osteopathy" than those in the U.S. Ten-fingered osteopathy is the area of osteopathy that can help address most common back ailments through a hands-on approach, also known as osteopathic manipulative treatment or OMT.

When you visit an osteopath specializing in OMT for the first time, a detailed case history will be taken. In addition to reviewing past events, it's important to try to describe your current pain and loss of function as well as you can. Listening is one of the practitioner's greatest tools, and the clearer your version of the problem, the better. And remember those lists!

Next, you'll be examined. You might be asked to remove some of your clothes and put on a gown to make assessment and treatment easier, but not in all cases. During the first part of the examination, the osteopath will watch you in different postures—standing, sitting—and basic movements like walking and bending in different directions. This will reveal a huge amount of information that he or she can use in the hands-on part of the proceedings.

The osteopath will then use a highly developed sense of touch, called palpation, to find and analyze points of weakness or strain. You may be standing at first, or sitting, and then usually you will be lying on a treatment table like the ones used for massage. If your problem is back pain, the osteopath will gently feel and move the different structures in your back to figure out how best to treat you.

Then the fun starts. The techniques used by osteopaths include very gentle hold/release work, massage, stretching, gentle mobilizing of joints in your spine, shoulders, hips, knees, etc., and also manipulation. Manipulation is manual pressure on the spine, soft tissues, and nearby structures including the head and pelvis. Some people who haven't had manipulation before can get a little nervous about this process, but they should relax. Osteopaths are trained to manipulate just the right stuff. They might use gentle release techniques like craniosacral therapy (which we'll talk about in the next section), as they often do with children or anyone who will respond best to gentle handling, or they might opt for more dramatic thrusting techniques.

You might be lying on your back with a pillow on your chest and your arms folded across it as your practitioner rolls you and then thrusts, or you might be sitting up with your fingers laced together behind your neck and the osteopath's arms wrapped around your torso in what appears to be a bad dance move. Don't freak out, it's nothing personal. They're just trying to reestablish your body's structural and functional soundness.

Osteopaths can mobilize joints, relieve muscle spasms, and guide any number of structures back into alignment. As this happens, you might hear what sounds like cracking, clicking, or popping, but once again, don't panic! This is not the sound of your bones breaking. Those noises are generally considered to be the release and popping of nitrogen bubbles that build up in affected joints, like when you "crack" your knuckles. Doing this too often can cause hypermobility in the ligaments, so your goal should be not to rely on treatment more frequently than is healthy.

Then it will be your turn to listen. After your treatment, the osteopath will usually give you advice about posture, exercise, and work habits, to prevent your pain from returning. This might be the most crucial part of your visit. Don't let all of that palpation and manipulation go to waste. Things were put right and now it's your job to keep them right.

First thing to remember right after a session is to keep warm so your muscles don't go back into spasm. You can have a fabulous treatment and then head out into a cold, windy day and everything will tense up just like it was before you went in. So if it's cold or even a little cool, wrap yourself up. Then it's best if you rest your back by not doing anything stupid. This doesn't mean staying in bed and not moving around. Unless your practitioner has told you to, it's been proven to be better in most cases to keep up some movement while you're getting back to normal. Just don't carry groceries, or bend awkwardly, or go back to work and "relax" with your spine slumped over your desk. Take responsibility for your own recovery.

Because everyone with back trouble is different, the number of treatments you'll need varies from person to person. After your first visit, an osteopath will be able to give you an idea of how often you will need to return. For mild acute pain, often one or two treatments will do the trick, but some chronic conditions will need ongoing maintenance, like your twelve-year-old car.

You should be aware that too much manipulation isn't good for you, like cracking your knuckles over and over. If you have a recurring problem and you keep going back for the same sort of manipulative treatment, something is wrong. Manipulation that takes place too often over years and years can make muscles and ligaments sluggish and hard to heal. The point of professional treatment is not just short-term relief. You need to find a permanent solution to your back problem, so if one thing isn't working, try something different.

Usually you will feel much better after an osteopathic treatment, often right away. But there is a settling-down period, especially after vigorous manipulation, and the full benefits of a treatment won't be felt for twenty-four to forty-eight hours. So don't panic if you don't feel a lot better within the first few hours. Good things come to those who wait.

CRANIOSACRAL THERAPY

THE TERM "CRANIOSACRAL therapy" was coined in the 1970s by Dr. John Upledger, an American osteopath, but the practice itself goes back to the start of last century and a daring osteopath named William Sutherland. While perusing the bones in the human skull he could see that they were clearly "designed" to move. Back then, and to some extent even now, conventional medicine asserted that the bones of the skull were meant to form an immoveable sphere to encase the brain. Obviously this isn't true of newborns, who, after that fun-filled trip down the birth canal, frequently come out looking like one of the Coneheads. But it was thought that the bones in the skull of an adult are fused and fixed.

After years of experimenting on himself—bet he was a laugh at parties—Sutherland found this not to be true. He discovered that gentle manipulation of the bones in the skull could have profound physical effects. He also discovered something else. He detected a subtle, rhythmic movement emanating from the bones of the skull, which traveled down the spinal cord and from there through the rest of the body. Sutherland called it the Primary Respiratory Impulse because it felt similar to our breathing rhythm, but these days we just call it cranial rhythm or cranial motion as it has nothing to do with our breathing.

Cranial rhythm seems to flow through the cerebrospinal fluid and the system of membranes around the brain and spinal cord all the way down to the sacrum. (That's where "craniosacral" comes from.) The movement is actually a subtle but measurable expansion and contraction. Modern sophisticated brain scans (PET scans) have confirmed this rhythm within the brain. Sutherland believed cranial rhythm to be the essential life force or energy, which is somewhat similarly described in various Eastern belief systems as kundalini or chi.

The function of cranial rhythm seems to be to organize and regulate the flow of energy through the body, but of course like any physical system it can be damaged. Luckily, it can also be repaired.

More and more people with back and neck pain are finding relief through craniosacral therapy. You can either see a craniosacral therapist or an osteopath who has learned it as a basic part of osteopathic training. But be prepared for the most subtle form of treatment you have ever had.

Some craniosacral therapists will take the usual medical history and listen to you about your current symptoms. Others will get straight to the physical stuff, and actually "listen" with their hands. Either way, you'll eventually lie on an examination or massage table while the practitioner rests his or her hands on or under your head and different locations along your spine down to your tailbone. Then come the very subtle adjustments in the form of shifts and slight tilts of pressure. These movements are intended to release blockages and aid the flow of your cranial rhythm.

People with pain from car accidents or other traumatic injuries are often amazed at the relief they get from craniosacral therapy, especially after trying everything else that conventional medicine has to offer. Craniosacral treatments often come hot on the heels of desperation. Many are pleasantly surprised.

The head, neck, and lower back are especially prone to disturbances of cranial rhythms from injury, but apparently treatments can help with a wide variety of ailments. Among the most successfully treated patients are babies with colic. The theory is that organs, including the stomach, could have been adversely affected by that rather stressful trip down the birth canal mentioned before. It's also possible that the effects of a forceps delivery on a baby's fragile skull can lead to headaches or other problems. Nerves that run through openings in the skull and the rest of the spine determine organ function and can be especially vulnerable to undue twisting and compression. Sometimes just a few minutes of treatment can fix up an infant who has been suffering for months.

There are a lot of skeptics out there who doubt the effectiveness of craniosacral therapy or even the idea that cranial rhythm exists. But the number of people who have been cured of both chronic and acute pain is growing. It's hard to believe in a psychosomatic response from a six-month-old child.

PHYSICAL THERAPY

PHYSICAL THERAPISTS (PTs) ARE very user-friendly practitioners for people with back trouble, although they can deal with a wide array of physical ailments. Their goal is pain relief and the restoration of function through natural, physical means. What distinguishes them from a lot of other practitioners is a practical emphasis on rehabilitation and prevention through exercise and education.

You might be referred to a physical therapist through your GP or another doctor, or you might work with one in hospital as part of rehabilitation. But you don't need a referral to see one, unless your insurance coverage requires it. In any case, the PT will take a history of your injury and any other relevant details, and then observe as you go through a series of movements that will give further clues about the nature of your problem. They'll be looking at the strength and length of your muscles, joint mobility, and overall function—what you can do and how you do it.

Once the problem is identified, your PT will discuss a treatment program with you that usually involves several steps.

There's heat therapy, which means using an infrared lamp directed at your back while you lie on a table and dream of winning gold in the Olympics. Heat helps your muscles relax by increasing circulation and oxygenating the affected area. Sometimes releasing the muscle spasm in this way alone is enough to get rid of or greatly reduce your pain.

Physical therapists also use massage and soft-tissue mobilization, as well as more vigorous manipulation as described earlier. Then there's always one of their many wonderful electromechanical devices. PTs have some amazing equipment in their arsenal, each piece cleverly designed to relieve your pain, decrease swelling, and enhance healing. Ultrasound is commonly used, and comes in the form of a wand emitting sound waves that humans can't hear. The PT rubs it over the surface of your skin, which has been prepared with lubricant conducting gel, and the waves penetrate tissue to a depth of about two inches. This causes a series of reactions including heat. Blood and lymphatic circulation is heightened, and muscle spasms and pain are interrupted. The treatment is extremely pleasant.

Then there's transcutaneous electrical nerve stimulation, more casually known as TENS. They put some of that gel on the skin of your back, and then apply these little electrical pads, usually two on each side of the spine. The pads are connected by wires to a battery-powered stimulator that can be adjusted for strength, frequency, and length of pulse. The sensation is like tiny little pinpricks on and just below the surface of the skin, but it's not painful. Just a little weird. It works in the same way that acupuncture does, by stimulating nerves and triggering the release of chemicals in the brain and spinal cord that block pain. TENS really just relieves symptoms, and shouldn't be seen as a cure, but when your condition is unremitting, any relief is welcome and therapeutic.

Although it's not used as much as it used to be, some physical therapists still see traction as an effective treatment for certain back conditions involving spinal compression. Traction has been used for thousands of years and, no matter how they dress it up, it still looks like a form of medieval torture. But it can actually feel great. You lie on a special table or bed with a harness around your lower torso and another one around your pelvis. Then these harnesses are very gently (mechanically) pulled in opposite directions. The point is to stretch muscles and joints, and reduce pressure on discs and nerves.

There are other devices and techniques that physical therapists use to treat pain, but in keeping with the importance they place on education, they can also help reeducate your muscles. The way they do this is through various electrical biofeedback devices attached to the affected area that can actually tell you with visual or aural signals when you're moving the right way or not.

After you've had a range of treatments, there's usually more education, but this time your brain needs to be a little more actively engaged than it was while your muscles got a workout. This is when the PT will teach you, often using models and charts, how your back works and why you ended up in pain. Pay attention. It helps to be able to visualize what goes on inside when you're trying to be good to your back. At this point you might be given or prescribed a corset or support of some kind to help you in the early stages of recovery. Just don't rely on these. What you really need is exercise and that's what's coming next. You'll get a series of exercises to do, specifically tailored to your individual problems and abilities. Remember that the best chance you have to avoid pain in the future is to follow good advice.

Occasionally, certain conditions might best respond to exercise in water, also called hydrotherapy. Physical therapists trained in hydrotherapy can devise a program that will decompress your spine, strengthen your muscles, mobilize your joints, improve circulation, induce relaxation, and relieve pain, all while you're flopping around in a heated pool. Nice work if you can get it. But take it seriously and stick with it. Exercising in water is one of those things that can really help you maintain a healthy back, and because it's very low impact, it's particularly good to do as you get older, and older . . .

CHIROPRACTIC

Chiropractic therapy was developed by Daniel David Palmer in 1895. Like his osteopathic counterpart, he was searching for natural, alternative treatments for pain and disease, and came up with a system largely based on manipulation.

A chiropractor's approach to your condition is similar to an osteopath's, but there are some significant differences. He or she will first take a full medical history followed by an examination and more often than not will order X-rays. In fact chiropractors order X-rays five times more frequently than osteopaths because they use them as fundamental diagnostic tools. Chiropractors believe that the manipulation they do is relevant only for joint and other structural dysfunctions, which X-rays can tell them. Often they have their own X-ray facility in their office.

While their brand of manipulation has many things in common with aspects of osteopathy, their style is somewhat different. When they examine you, they will look for areas of "subluxation"—a joint, usually a spinal one, that isn't quite where it's supposed to be. Subluxation disturbs blood flow and affects nerve roots, not just to the muscles and bones but the organs as well, and manipulation is designed to correct this.

Often chiropractors will favor quick thrusts and will work on surrounding soft tissue to an extent, but they largely focus on the spine and its associated structures. They will also occasionally use some of the electronic equipment such as TENS favored by physical therapists.

Like other back-care professionals, chiropractors will give you advice about posture and exercise. Be sure to heed their words. They've seen a lot more bad backs than you have and will know what works to keep pain from coming back!

ORTHOPEDICS

ORTHOPEDIC CONSULTANTS OR orthopedic surgeons are the medical specialists who look after the musculoskeletal system. To see one, you'll need a referral from your GP, unless you meet one through the emergency room of your local hospital. Orthopedic consultants are the doctors you go to when you've had broken bones or other severe trauma caused, for example, by a sporting or car accident. Or, you've tried every other form of back treatment and are considering surgery.

While most of them have no background in "alternative" or "complementary" therapies, they have over a dozen years of medical training and tons of experience dealing with all sorts of stresses to bones, joints, ligaments, tendons, muscles, and nerves. The term "orthopedic" used to apply to doctors devoted to children with skeletal disorders, but now they care for everyone. Because they're attached to hospitals, orthopedic surgeons have access to an impressive selection of high-tech diagnostic and therapeutic equipment. If you become one of their patients, you'll find they start out like every other practitioner, by listening.

The first step with an orthopedic surgeon is the taking of a medical history. And don't be shy about bringing out your lists. Even though the person sitting across the desk from you may have spent more time at university than you have in a job, like all health practitioners they'll still get their most important information from you, and they'll appreciate you helping to make their job easier. Then comes the physical examination, which may be either followed or preceded by blood tests, X-rays, or scans.

The type of treatment you get depends on what's wrong. You may get off light—with some counseling, medication, and instructions for exercise. Or the recommendation might be for surgery. It's important to know that back surgery is performed much less frequently than it used to be, and even orthopedic surgeons see it as a last resort after you have explored a lot of other options. In the U.S., less than 1 percent of back pain sufferers need surgery. It will only be considered if your pain is debilitating and chronic, and if your particular problem is the sort that historically responds well to surgery.

People who suffer from persistent sciatica caused by a prolapsed disc are likely candidates, and indeed this is the most common "back" operation performed. Often, the symptoms will include constant pain, progressive loss of feeling or muscle function, or even the much-dreaded loss of bowel or bladder control. The disc is usually in the lower lumbar area, and it will either be removed completely, or the nasty bit will be trimmed. This is called a diskectomy. Or, pain might be triggered by part of the facet bone pressing on a nerve root, and the surgeon will remove the offending piece of bone. This is called—wait for it—a facetectomy. Those medical guys are real poets. Another common procedure is called "spinal fusion," which is indicated when there's too much movement between vertebrae that is causing serious problems, and the surgeon fuses them together. Surgery may also be recommended in certain cases of spinal stenosis.

Obviously surgery is the most invasive treatment possible, and should only be considered when your other options have run out. In the old days, people who had back surgery stayed in bed for months, but now most patients get up and walk around within days of an operation, and there will usually be a course of physiotherapy that you need to follow if you want full mobility. It's crucial to follow your surgeon's advice about when to return to work, but generally, light activity is going to speed your recovery. Just don't be incredibly dumb and go bowling.

RHEUMATOLOGY

A RHEUMATOLOGIST IS a medical doctor who specializes in conditions marked by inflammation and pain in the joints, muscles, and fibrous tissues, like arthritis. You'll need a referral to see a rheumatologist, and he or she will take the usual medical history and perform an examination.

Treatment will often include physiotherapy and exercise, as well as anti-inflammatory medication and referral to another specialist when necessary. There have been some recent significant breakthroughs in the treatment of rheumatoid arthritis, many involving diet and the use of over-the-counter supplements. But always consult your doctor and read up on the subject in more depth yourself before going on a spending spree in your local health food store.

ACUPUNCTURE

ACUPUNCTURE IS A healing technique developed over five thousand years ago, and since then has been used as a fundamental medical treatment in China, Japan, and Tibet. According to its traditional practitioners, acupuncture is an effective treatment for almost every ailment we can have because it stimulates the mind to heal the body by balancing the yin and yang energy flow. It is so effective as a way to block pain that acupuncture is commonly used in China as the primary anesthetic during surgery. Although it's now heartily embraced in Western society, and often medical doctors will suggest it as a treatment for pain, they usually believe acupuncture's effectiveness stops there.

The first part of the consultation will involve careful questioning and observation by the practitioner, to determine the exact nature of your disharmony. So even if you came in complaining about your bad back, you'll be asked about lifestyle, diet, circulation, sleep patterns, and your emotional state. You'll also have your tongue examined and your pulse felt. The quality, strength, and rhythm of your pulse will reveal a lot to an acupuncturist, who will decide on treatment accordingly. This is a very holistic approach. The idea is that symptoms don't exist in isolation, but emerge from interconnected systems.

In ancient times they used sharpened stones, and later on, needles carved from bone and bamboo, but now acupuncturists use sterile steel, silver, or gold needles. The needles are inserted for a second or two, or left in place for up to thirty minutes depending on your condition. After insertion, the needles are usually rotated. Along the meridians or energy pathways used as a guide, there are over seven hundred points on your body where the needles can be inserted. The effect can be anything from a heavy ache to relaxation and the complete relief of pain. Some patients report feeling like their body is lit up like an electronic circuit board. This is a very successful acupuncture session.

Western medical experts say that all this happens because the insertion of the needles stimulates the release of hormones (including endorphins and enkephalins) in the brain and spinal cord, blocking the pain. Traditional practitioners will explain it in a more holistic way. The important thing is that most patients will get relief from pain, and maybe even more.

You can get almost immediate results from acupuncture, but it usually requires more than one visit. Sometimes it will just take a couple of treatments, but more often there is some relief of symptoms after five or so visits. Deep-seated problems can take months to address.

For some patients who are uncomfortable with needle-insertion, some acupuncturists are now using lasers to stimulate the same points along the meridians. This is more expensive but just as effective.

Many practitioners of acupuncture also practice TCM

(traditional Chinese medicine), which involves herbal treatments for various conditions from headaches to period pain to liver stress to chronic fatigue syndrome. Don't be put off by the smells if they suggest you boil up a strange tea using fresh herbs, some of which you've never even heard of! In conjunction with the acupuncture, TCM can be amazingly effective.

MASSAGE

IN WESTERN SOCIETY, massage was seen for a long time as merely a soothing, comforting technique that at best alleviated symptoms like pain and spasms. But older cultures such as those in China, Japan, India, Greece, and Rome have long appreciated its fantastic remedial properties. Finally, the rest of the world is catching on.

Of course like all other practitioners, the degree of skill and sensitivity as well as the individual technique varies enormously from one massage therapist to another. Some seem to think they're slapping around a dead fish while others have a true gift for healing. A really good massage can not only make your pain go away, it can help keep it away, especially when accompanied by the sound exercise and lifestyle advice that a lot of massage therapists dispense these days.

Private health funds have recognized that massage is a valuable tool in overall health maintenance, and it's often less expensive in the long run than other therapies that might do the same thing. This is why most funds will now partially reimburse you for visits to registered massage therapists. But even if you can't get any cash back, you will be getting one of the most relaxing and pleasurable forms of treatment there is.

Obviously it's always nice to have a massage, but if you have back or neck pain caused by muscle tightness, cramping, or other health problems like bronchitis, a massage can be heavenly. Just make sure you explain the nature of your injury or strain to the therapist, as well as any other treatment you're getting, as this will determine the type of massage you're given.

The therapist might start by using heated towels or a heat lamp to warm up your back before moving it around. This will help your muscles and your mind relax. Next is the application of massage oil or cream, often scented with an essential oil that can help the relaxing–healing process along.

There are dozens of types of massage, from mild Swedish, which focuses on loosening the muscles, to shiatsu, which uses pressure exerted on meridian points, sort of like acupuncture without the needles. Most massage therapists will use a combination of techniques depending on their own inclinations and your needs. This can include rubbing, stroking, kneading, pounding, slapping, and vibrating. They can use their hands, their elbows, and even their knees. And of course there are those who will actually walk on your back, but if you have back trouble, this is probably not the way to go.

One of the most satisfying branches of massage is **reflexology**. For many thousands of years, healers in China, India, and Egypt have recognized that points of congestion and tension in different parts of the feet and hands mirror congestion and tension in corresponding parts of the body. By stimulating and massaging these points on the feet and hands, the distant affected body parts are stimulated and healed. As we've been saying all along, sometimes it's very hard to determine the exact origin of pain that manifests itself in our backs. Often it will actually be referred from organs like the liver or uterus, and when the right buttons are pushed by a massage therapist who knows reflexology, the result can be extraordinary.

Another effective technique used by massage therapists for the treatment of back pain is cupping. This is an ancient Chinese remedy that has marvelous instantaneous effects. Making sure your skin is lubricated with oil or gel, the therapist will light a flame and hold it in or under a specially designed small glass cup with rounded edges. The heat will create a vacuum inside the cup that's then placed on the area of your back that is in pain or spasm. You will feel a sucking effect on your soft tissues, and while it's not unpleasant, it can occasionally be a little bit painful. But it's worth it. Usually, the therapist will prepare and place several cups around different spots on your back. They might be left in place for a time, or they might be gently dragged across the surface of the skin, massaging as they go. Cupping like this is sort of massage in reverse, and it has an amazing ability to undo muscle spasms. It's also extremely effective if you have a lung infection, and seems to loosen congestion and unblock your airways. When the cups are left in place for a time, they can cause slight bruising, but this will fade like any other bruise.

Massage does a lot more than you might imagine. In addition to making you feel wonderfully relaxed if not downright euphoric, it increases lymphatic and blood circulation. This means that oxygen and other nutrients get delivered more quickly and efficiently to cells that need them to heal. Also, by-products of damaged cells in the form of acids are dissolved and carried away faster. We tend to forget that, while back pain might feel like a large phenomenon, damage occurs chemically on a cellular level. Massage will stimulate faster cell recovery and help deliver you from pain.

Massage also enhances muscle elasticity and tone. It is curative and preventative, and works really well in conjunction with other treatments such as physiotherapy, chiropractic, and osteopathy when manipulation has been used.

A fairly recent development in massage therapy is what is known as the office massage. This is often given at an office or place of work by therapists who have been hired by enlightened management, or just by individuals in the company who recognize the value of on-the-job treatments. These massages are given while you sit in a chair, fully clothed, and the therapist works on your back, neck, and head. It takes about the same time as your average coffee break and is a hell of a lot better for you. It's just the thing for those of us who spend obscene amounts of time sitting at desks, glued to our computer keyboards, wondering why we get headaches, stiff necks, and lower back pain.

ROLFING

ROLFING IS A holistic method of soft tissue manipulation developed by Dr. Ida P. Rolf over fifty years ago. Her system, which she called structural integration, is based on the idea of reshaping and reorganizing the body so that it works with gravity rather than against it.

Rolfing addresses the fascial connections of the body to enhance movement, relax muscles, improve posture, and ease blood flow.

Years ago, the technique was more vigorous than it is now, and many patients complained of painful treatments. All that has changed, and although Rolfing still involves quite deep manipulation and massage, the methods have been refined and you are much more likely to have your pain reduced rather than increased.

Rolfing can be effective in relieving acute and chronic pain, and has been very successful at correcting structural dysfunctions such as extreme lordosis.

KINESIOLOGY AND TOUCH FOR HEALTH

IN THE EARLY 1960s, a chiropractor named George Goodheart (nice name for a health practitioner) developed a simple but original way of working with muscles. He realized that weak muscles can cause opposing healthy muscles to tighten up. So instead of just working to relieve a spasm on one side, he suggested strengthening the muscle on the other side, or the spasm would keep coming back. Makes sense.

Another chiropractor named John Thie, who had worked with Goodheart, expanded these principles using the muscles themselves as biofeedback tools in conjunction with our bodies' electromagnetic energy system. This is the same as the system used in acupuncture, where energy flows along what are identified as meridians. Thie's system of muscle testing simply involves the practitioner touching the area where the patient's muscle engages in order to determine the effectiveness of that muscle and the flow of energy along associated meridians. He called it "Touch for Health." This incredibly basic diagnostic tool can be used to help the body heal itself. The system, with some variations, is also called kinesiology. While advocates of the technique claim that it actually works on the whole body based on its interconnectedness, it is especially suited to people with ongoing back strain where soft tissues including muscles are affected.

The treatment is as simple as the diagnosis, and is called muscle balancing. All it involves is gentle hand or finger pressure on the meridian point that is associated with the weakness causing pain. The length of time the pressure is maintained depends on the severity of the problem.

Touch for Health sounds so simple that it may be difficult to believe it works. But many sufferers have found that long-standing problems disappear overnight. And if you're like most people, you won't care how someone helps relieve you of your pain, as long as they do it!

PODIATRY

PODIATRY WAS CALLED chiropody until the late 1970s, when they changed it because people kept getting chiropodists confused with chiropractors. Technically speaking, podiatrists are foot doctors. They can deal with any problems of the feet from athlete's foot to ingrown toenails to more serious structural dysfunctions like fallen arches. But another exciting thing they can do is treat your bad back. It depends on your condition, of course, but there are certain lower back disorders that are actually the ugly by-products of a dysfunctional gait or structural abnormalities stemming from the feet.

As we keep reminding you, the human body is an integrated system, and what happens at one end can have serious consequences at the other end. If you have a right foot that rolls outward when you walk, it's going to push your right hip upward. This will have a ripple effect and eventually your whole pelvis is involved and you might have chronic sciatica. You may have visited other kinds of doctors and therapists for years, and the symptoms go away for a while, only to return after the effects of a treatment wear off.

Like other practitioners, good podiatrists will take your medical history, but they'll also measure the bones in your legs to make sure you aren't suffering merely from a difference in length. And then they'll get you to do something you probably haven't done before. Often they'll get you to walk on a treadmill in bare feet while they video you. If there's a significant problem with your gait a podiatrist will see it right away, or he or she might analyze the videotape later to break down your movements into component parts, making for an easier assessment. The great news is that if there is a problem with your feet that's causing back pain, a podiatrist can usually correct it.

The way the podiatrist does this is by fitting you with a pair of customized orthotics. We're not talking about those little flaps you can buy at sports stores that you slip into your running shoes. We're talking about high-tech, hard plastic devices. First your podiatrist takes molds of your feet, and then orders a pair of slim plastic platforms in the shape of your feet created by a lab that will be sent your exact specifications. The podiatrist then shapes the orthotics to compensate for your particular mechanical dysfunction. Even if you only have one tricky foot, you'll need orthotics for both feet because the platform will add height, and you don't want an uneven stance. Of course orthotics can also compensate for uneven leg length.

It may seem like an odd way to solve a back problem, but sometimes you need to look beyond the obvious.

MAGNETIC FIELD THERAPY

THE THEORY BEHIND magnetic field therapy is that our blood contains iron and potassium, which, in red blood cells, can be drawn to the affected area by magnets. This concentration is meant to increase lymphatic drainage, therefore it enhances healing and decreases pain. Proximity to magnets is achieved in a number of ways, such as lying on a table implanted with magnets, or wearing magnetized belts.

Although studies are inconclusive, there is some evidence that treatment with magnets can relieve symptoms of fibromyalgia and other kinds of back pain.

NUTRITION

MORE AND MORE research is pointing to diet as a contributing factor in back pain caused by a variety of diseases, including fibromyalgia, and forms of arthritis including ankylosing spondylitis. You can do a lot of reading yourself, but it may be easier to visit a nutritionist or general practitioner who is aware of the connection between allergens and inflammatory conditions, as well as other nutritional factors that can affect your back.

Here again we're reminded of how integrated the body's systems are. You really can't separate one from the other. Especially when you're looking for a solution that is proving elusive. Sometimes sensitivities to foods like wheat and dairy can cause problems in the joints. So an altered diet might be recommended, as well supplements such as fish oils. Toxins including cigarettes, alcohol, and coffee are usually off the menu for people with inflammatory problems, but you won't know to what extent all this clean living will get rid of your pain until you try it, will you?

Some studies show that people with fibromyalgia often have magnesium deficiencies, and there is certainly a connection between lack of magnesium and muscle spasms as well as fatigue. You may want to take a magnesium supplement, but as the dosage will vary according to the severity of your condition, it's good to be guided by someone who knows what he or she is doing.

Magnesium deficiency can result in increased susceptibility to aluminum toxicity, which is also associated with fibromyalgia. A substance that naturally occurs in the body, called malic acid, can be a good aluminum detoxifier, and taken as a supplement together with magnesium might be just the cocktail you need to banish pain. Manganese and vitamin B1 have also been proven to help people struggling with back pain.

NATUROPATHY

To get a different perspective on your back problem and also learn about a variety of supplements that can help you cope with pain, you could visit a good naturopath. Like other practitioners, naturopaths will take a medical history and suggest a range of treatments and therapies, but their approach is definitely holistic. In other words, they'll look at all of your symptoms, including habits, diet, stress, build, and not just your back pain. They will try to treat the causes of your condition, not merely their effects.

The good thing about consulting a naturopath is that he or she can recommend healthy, effective supplements in doses specially tailored to your needs. They might suggest an amino acid like diphenylalanine or they might mix up a combination of herbs that are known to diminish pain and other symptoms of back trouble. Or, if you suffer from any arthritic condition, they can recommend a whole other range of supplements, from vitamin and mineral therapy to herbs.

Similar treatments are available in health food shops, but the manufacturers of these supplements usually just recommend the absolute minimum dosage, so you may be taking something (and spending a lot of money) for months and think the stuff is no good because it has had no effect.

Naturopathy is no less an exact science than orthopedics. If you're going to go with a natural alternative, make sure you get advice from an expert. If naturopaths can't help you, or they need more diagnostic information from blood tests or ultrasounds, they will refer you to the appropriate medical doctor or complementary practitioner.

HOMEOPATHY

AS WITH ALL remedial disciplines, the effectiveness of homeopathy depends on the skill of the individual practitioner. What good homeopaths do is listen carefully to your description of all of your symptoms—not just the fact that your back has been acting up—as well as your emotional state. Then they'll figure out which substance can cause the same range of symptoms, and administer it in highly diluted form that you take as drops under the tongue.

For example, you may have a cold that has the same symptoms as mercury poisoning, so your remedy will be a tiny amount of mercury diluted in water. Homeopathy works in a similar way to conventional treatments for allergies or to vaccines where a small dose of a substance actually protects against it by getting the body to fight the problem itself. Once you start taking the remedy, you should notice an improvement within a day or two. If not, you're on the wrong remedy and you should stop.

Homeopathy is practiced worldwide, and has long been popular among England's royal family, and millions of others not normally associated with "alternative" therapies. Part of the appeal of homeopathic medicine is that it is safe, nonaddictive, fast-working, and cheap (although that last point probably wasn't the main selling point to the royals). Best of all, it works. Just don't expect to walk into your local health food shop and buy an over-the-counter homeopathic remedy that seems to address your symptoms. The right remedy will more likely be found by a trained professional who will ask questions you wouldn't even have thought to ask.

BOWEN TECHNIQUE

THIS AMAZINGLY SIMPLE, noninvasive technique was developed by an Australian named Tom Bowen in the 1950s, and although he never explained how it worked—maybe he wasn't sure himself!—he taught other practitioners how to do it, and the practice has spread around the world.

There is no diagnostic phase of your visit to a Bowen practitioner. Instead, the treatment is the same no matter what your complaint, but it does seem to be especially effective with people who suffer from back and neck pain. What happens is that you lie on a mat on the floor while the therapist uses thumbs and fingers to gently touch or squeeze certain points on your body, often at or near the joints. One of the key elements of Bowen technique is that this point-squeezing has to be done in a predetermined sequence. A session lasts for between forty-five minutes and an hour, and during that time, the practitioner will leave the room a couple of times. But it isn't something you said. These little intervals are intended to let your body absorb the effects of the treatment.

In some cases, persistent pain can be relieved right away or in a few sessions. Other times, it takes longer. But how does it work? The theory is that the technique corrects energy imbalances through subtle soft tissue releases. Another theory is that it works on the points where nerves exit from fascial openings. Whatever the secret, Bowen Technique works for a lot of people.

A further refinement of Bowen Technique is called vibro-muscular harmonization technique, which builds on the work Bowen was doing before he died in 1982. It employs the same basic set of moves but has added a lot more of the squeezey parts. Practitioners say that this advanced technique gets quicker and more consistent results.

HYPNOSIS

BECAUSE BACK PAIN is so often related to mental or emotional stress, and indeed the way we deal with stress, some people have found relief through hypnotherapy. A study conducted by the U.S. National Institute of Health concluded that hypnosis can be useful in easing chronic pain. The idea is that your sensitivity to pain, and the way you react to it (which may be out of proportion to your injury), can be blunted.

Hypnosis can also have positive effects by enhancing how we feel or think about ourselves and our problems.

PAIN CLINICS

IN SOME VERY rare cases, back pain may not go away with either conventional or unconventional treatments. When pain is constant or repetitive for a period longer than three months, it is called chronic pain. Victims of this sort of pain may be unable to work or even live a normal life, and virtually all aspects of their lives are affected, often resulting in relationship breakdowns, depression, and deterioration of general health. Fortunately there is good news even for them.

In most large cities, hospitals now have pain clinics where numerous therapists and doctors including psychologists, MDs, specialists, occupational therapists, or physiotherapists work in a team to help patients manage severe chronic pain in a variety of ways. In very rare cases where this multipronged approach has limited success, patients might be involved in trials of new medication, and others might be implanted with something called a dorsal column stimulator. These are very costly, and while they can mask the pain for a while, the effect usually wears off. There are also devices called intrathecal pumps that can be implanted in the abdomen. They store a reservoir of a painkilling drug, such as morphine, which is delivered straight to the spinal cord so that the negative side effects are minimized.

All chronic pain management programs include psychological training sessions, where patients learn how to change their behavior and the way they think of and deal with their pain. This isn't a quick fix or an easy cure, but it can work, and helps the patient reduce or eliminate his or her dependency on drugs and various mechanical supports including wheelchairs.

Progress is being made all the time in the treatment of chronic pain, but as always, the most important factor is the full, willing, educated participation of the sufferer.

• • •

There are some additional professional practices like the Alexander technique and Feldenkrais that have therapeutic properties, but their emphasis is actually more on maintenance and prevention, so we'll get to them in a later section.

DIAGNOSTIC TOOLS

A **range of practitioners,** including GPs, orthopedic surgeons, osteopaths, chiropractors, and rheumatologists can order a variety of tests to help them accurately diagnose your back problem. We thought it might be useful for you to know a little bit about how the tests work and what they can tell us—so that when a practitioner says, "I'm going to order some tests," and then starts scribbling on a pad, you're not left wishing you had studied harder at school.

It's also important to understand that sophisticated imaging techniques like CAT scans and MRIs may reveal little when it comes to many forms of back pain. So if you feel a small twinge when you wake up, don't go rushing off to your practitioner demanding a series of wildly expensive tests. In many cases of back pain, your own body will tell you and your doctor more than all the fancy tests can.

BLOOD TESTS

A PRACTITIONER MAY order a blood test for a variety of reasons. Your white blood cell count will indicate whether your immune system has been activated, so it can rule out a number of diseases. Or there may be a possibility that you're suffering from an inflammatory condition with rheumatoid factors. In the latter, a certain kind of white blood cell will show up, and although around eight percent of healthy people also have these cells but don't have the inflammatory disease, if you've got other symptoms there's a pretty good chance you have it.

Blood tests can also reveal levels of hormones such as estrogen, cortisone, and thyroxine to determine, among other things, the presence of diseases including osteoporosis. Remember, in terms of results, "positive" means you've got something that is a cause of concern and is not a good thing.

X-RAYS

AN X-RAY IS an electromagnetic ray that can penetrate soft tissue to varying degrees and be projected onto a screen or film to produce a photograph. It can show the outline of various organs like the heart and lungs, and when the patient is injected with dyes it can also show blood vessels, but primarily it's used to show the bones. An X-ray cannot clearly show what's happening with discs, nerves, muscles, tendons, or the lymphatic system, although in some cases the conditions of some of these tissues can be inferred. X-rays can reveal the approximate degree of bone density, arthritis, cancer, and many other diseases. Even so, when it comes to bad backs, probably more X-rays are taken than need to be.

As with any investigation regarding your health, find out why your practitioner is asking for an X-ray. As long as you're not being X-rayed repeatedly, the chance of harm from radiation is very small.

CAT SCANS

ALSO KNOWN AS CT (Computed Tomography) scans, CAT (Computerized Axial Tomography) scans are X-rays that pass through the patient's body at various angles from a machine mounted within a big, fat, space-age-looking tube that you've probably seen on *ER* or in movies. The patient lies down on a platform that is conveyed into the open-ended tube so pictures can be taken.

After the pictures are taken, a computer layers them, creating a three-dimensional, cross-sectional view. This gives a more distinct image of the spine's internal structures, including some details of the discs. A CAT scan can even show a disc pressing on the spinal cord or a nerve root. Osteoporosis and spinal stenosis can also be detected this way.

MAGNETIC RESONANCE IMAGING (MRI) SCANS

OUTWARDLY RESEMBLING THE CAT scanner, an MRI scanner is also a tube that surrounds the patient on a guided platform, but instead of projected X-rays, it uses powerful electromagnets built into the tube, which cover the patient in a magnetic field. Sounds like science fiction, doesn't it? Well it gets better.

Our bodies contain abundant amounts of hydrogen, and when the magnetic field excites our hydrogen atoms, they transmit faint radio signals. These signals are then converted by a computer into highly detailed images that include nerves, ligaments, and discs inside bony structures.

As with CAT scanners, people sometimes get a little claustrophobic inside the tube. So that the pictures can be clear, you're not supposed to move at all! And the surface you're lying on is pretty hard. But the outcome can be worth it.

MRI is safer than X-rays because there's no radiation and of course it can tell us a lot more, but it doesn't always tell us everything. As with regular X-rays and CAT scans, what it reveals doesn't always correlate with the patient's symptoms. This is another reminder that what we call the back can't be broken down into isolated parts, but is instead composed of a system so integrated with the rest of the body that sometimes the cause of the problem eludes us.

ULTRASOUND SCANS

AS A DIAGNOSTIC tool, ultrasound can generate images that distinguish between different tissues inside the body. From these pictures that come up live on a monitor (like a TV screen), we can also measure and assess different structures and detect movement.

First a radiographer or radiologist puts lubricating gel on your skin. Then he or she holds the horizontal bar that emits inaudible sound waves with a frequency of over 20,000 cycles per second onto the area to be investigated, and drags it across your skin. Bone and air in the body reflect most of the sound waves, while other tissues absorb or reflect the waves to varying degrees. The image we see on the screen is the shape of the sound waves' echo.

Although it's not as detailed as an MRI, ultrasound imagery is particularly useful in the analysis of certain soft tissue and joint problems.

PET SCANS

PET IS SHORT for positron emission tomography or photon emission tomography, which is why it is easier just to say

PET scans. Radioisotopes are injected into the bloodstream and then a gamma camera flashes gamma rays (we know, it sounds so Star Trek), which can detect areas of increased cellular activity, sometimes related to conditions like rheumatoid arthritis, fractures, infection, and bone cancers.

5 DRUGS

The **purpose of** drugs in back care is often pain relief. There are two main types of drugs you might take for back pain: analgesics, which are purely for pain relief, and anti-inflammatories, which, you guessed it, reduce inflammation and associated pain.

ANALGESICS

THE MOST WIDELY used analgesic is acetaminophen, which can deal with mild pain. They now sell slow-release tablets, so you can take fewer pills but get the same dosage. Acetaminophen is available over-the-counter in any super-market or pharmacy. You can also get acetaminophen mixed with codeine, but it must be prescribed for you by a doctor. Acetaminophen on its own is safe for kids for a short time, but you should be wary of giving them codeine even in small doses, as it's hard on their young livers.

The thing to watch with codeine is that it can make you constipated. This is not what you want when you have a bad back, as straining on the toilet and any unwanted internal pressure can put a terrible load on your lower back and make the pain worse. So if you're taking codeine, drink tons of water, eat fruit, and avoid foods that tend to constipate, like french fries or anything fried. The water will also help flush the codeine through your liver. Remember that, like cigarettes, alcohol, heroin, and chocolate, codeine is addictive.

There are other over-the-counter pharmacy-only analgesics that contain an antihistamine/sedative called doxylamine succinate, which can be helpful when you have really severe pain, no prescription, and a lot of stress that may be contributing to muscle spasm and other tension. This is an adults-only drug, definitely not for kids under twelve. It may cause major drowsiness, so do not operate any heavy machinery—like a hairdryer—while you're taking it.

Then there are the analgesics that doctors can prescribe. These are stronger painkillers, also often mixed with acetaminophen. One of the most common is with codeine. Follow the prescribed dosage carefully and only take it if you have to. Same goes with dextropropoxyphene (Darvon) and dihydrocodeine (Synalgos). Sometimes it's good to try to take milder pain relievers during the day, and something stronger only before you go to bed to help you sleep and give your body a chance to relax and heal.

If your back pain is so bad that you've had to be carried into the emergency room at the local hospital, after assessing your condition they may administer Demerol, or even morphine, by injection or intravenous drip. Obviously these are last resort painkillers, and ones that should preferably be used only in the short term.

ANTI-INFLAMMATORIES

ANTI-INFLAMMATORY DRUGS reduce inflammation and also kill pain, so they're good for many forms of arthritis as well as any conditions that have caused inflammation and stiffness. Most anti-inflammatories are also called NSAIDs (non-steroidal anti-inflammatory drugs). The most popular of these is aspirin, but it can cause stomach upsets, internal bleeding, and even ringing in your ears if you take too much. A little easier on the tummy is another over-the-counter anti-inflammatory, ibuprofen, but it's still good to take it with food to minimize the chance of indigestion. If you have to take anti-inflammatories for a long time, you may also want to take another drug to protect your tummy. But adding drugs on drugs is generally not the best way to manage a problem.

There are stronger anti-inflammatories that your doctor can prescribe, such as diclofenac (Cataflam, Voltaren), keto-profen (Orudis, Oruvail), naproxen (Anaprox, Naprelan, Naprosyn, Aleve), and piroxicam (Feldene). Once again, you have to protect your digestive system, and if you're really experiencing trouble in that area, your doctor can always prescribe the drugs as suppositories. That will encourage you to find an alternative way to manage your pain.

Sometimes, if you have severe localized pain due to inflammation, your doctor may give you an injection of a strong anti-inflammatory steroid such as cortisone. Injected, it doesn't go through your stomach, so you don't get the negative side effects. Although this seems like you're only treating the symptom (the effects last for two to three hours and then your symptoms can return), often the pain retreats completely after about a day. Frequently, cortisone is administered with a little anesthetic to kill the pain immediately until the cortisone kicks in. Ideally, relief should last indefinitely if the cycle of inflammation is broken.

If you have persistent, severe sciatica, you might be given an epidural injection of an anti-inflammatory and anesthetic that goes straight into the membrane surrounding the spinal cord. This treatment is only administered after a really bad attack, and only if the pain isn't going away with other treatments.

MUSCLE RELAXANTS

THESE ARE AVAILABLE with a prescription, and are recommended only in cases of extreme muscle spasm. They'll temporarily turn you into The Blob on legs, so driving that forklift or even programming your VCR is definitely out. Sometimes releasing a spasm is enough to eliminate the problem that caused the pain, but usually muscle spasms have some structural source. So once the muscle relaxants have done their job, you need to solve the problem that made your muscles tighten up in the first place.

ALCOHOL

IN MODERATION—AND we really mean it—alcohol is a natural muscle relaxant and can help you unload stress. But in excess, alcohol is a really terrible treatment for your back. The problem is that in large quantities, it will severely dehydrate you, which is the worst thing you could do for muscles in spasm and strained ligaments. Alcohol constricts your blood vessels, too, and this is another way you'd be starving your tissues. You're delivering less fluid, less oxygen, and less nutrition to the areas that need all of those things to heal.

Also, when you've had a lot to drink and go to bed, you tend to lie there like a coma victim. That, and the loss of all those nutrients carried by the bloodstream, is why you will be even more stiff and sore the morning after than you were the night before.

OTHER DRUGS

In certain cases, drugs used for people with epilepsy can help control back pain, especially neuralgia, which feels like an electric shock that can run from the back down the legs, arms, and up the neck. Other severe chronic pain sufferers can be helped by some antidepressants, as the biochemical changes the pain has wrought on their central nervous systems are similar to those in the clinically depressed. In these cases, you need to talk to your doctor to determine the suitability of these treatments, and be very aware of side effects.

We haven't used any brand names here because we figure, why give the pharmaceutical companies free advertising? Also, it's always a good idea to ask your pharmacy for the generic version of a drug if there's no difference other than the lower price.

Obviously, with all drugs, read the labels and enclosed warnings before you take them and follow the instructions to the letter. Remember that drugs are not a cure. It's easy to forget that when you're in agony and then you take something and the agony goes away. The tendency is to think, well, that's taken care of. But of course it isn't. Unless you take responsibility for addressing the cause of your symptoms, that agony will be back. Don't make the mistake of getting on the pain–drugs–relief–pain–drugs–relief merry-go-round. That way lies addiction, a ruined stomach, screwed up liver and kidneys, poverty, depression, bad breath, B.O., loneliness, and death. Well, maybe we're exaggerating. It depends on your drug of choice. Just don't let yourself take what appears to be an easy option, when in the long run it's not an option at all.

6 DO-IT-YOURSELF BACK CARE

*A*s we've said, if you have symptoms of a serious back disorder, or back pain that doesn't go away after a few days, you should consult a back care practitioner. But what can you do yourself in the meantime? Plenty.

STOP AND REST

THE FIRST THING is to accept that your pain is a sign that something is wrong, so you should stop what you're doing and rest. This is really hard for some people who think that the world will end if they stop working/bench-pressing/vacuuming. Whatever it is you're doing, it's probably not curing cancer, so just let it go for a few days while you recover. And for you people out there who are curing cancer, even you need to stop what you're doing if your back acts up!

The best position to rest in is usually the one that feels most comfortable. It's not generally sitting or standing, as they promote spinal compression. That leaves lying down.

Sciatica and other back pain often fade when you lie on your back on a firm bed or couch, with a little support from a pillow or cushion or two under you knees. Or you can lie on the floor with your lower legs and feet resting on a chair or ottoman. And when we say lie down, we mean lie down flat. Don't have more then one pillow under your head, and don't put any under your shoulders or upper back. You can't look at this little hiatus as a way to get back into the daytime soaps. You need to be horizontal!

With disc problems, it's really important to stay horizontal as much as possible. Some people find that lying on their stomachs brings some relief. It can also help to then push up gently and slowly with the arms, while keeping the hips in contact with the floor.

And don't be an idiot. If you need assistance getting into or out of these positions and there's someone around who can lend a hand, accept it! There are times to be stoic, and times to be needy. This is the latter.

If you have a soft bed (very naughty—but more on that later) and you're having a bout of back pain, get a friend to put a board or an old door or something hard under the mattress until you can buy a firm one.

If you're not lying on your back, it's best to lie on the side that hurts less. Sometimes it relieves lower back pain to bring your knees up toward a fetal position. But wherever your knees are, put a cushion between them. This reduces the chance for your lower back and other structures like hips and pelvis to pull further out of alignment. Even after some people recover completely from pain, they continue to use a cushion between their knees in bed because it maintains good sleeping posture.

Handy hint number one—the most painless way to get out of bed is to roll on to your side and then push your torso up with your arms and hands as you swing your legs off the bed and let your feet touch the floor at the same time. Feel free to stop at a sitting position to let your back and neck adjust to what's happening. Then get up slowly using both legs equally, holding your abdominal muscles in. To get into bed, reverse the process. If you're lying on the floor, you can use the same technique, minus the leg swinging. In other words, don't let your back do any work it doesn't have to do.

Handy hint number two is for when your bad back happens to coincide with a cold. A lot of people make their injuries worse by "throwing" their backs further out when they sneeze or cough. Doing either of those things involves a huge amount of pressure and traumatic movement in your spine, so the next time you feel a sneeze or cough coming on, brace yourself by holding onto the back of a chair or a table or a door frame. It's amazing how much less impact your back will feel when you take your weight through your hands.

MOVE

DON'T LIE AROUND all day. At least every three hours you should try to get up and move around, just to keep your circulation going and your muscles happy. Use some common sense when it comes to the kind of movements you attempt. No matter how your injury or strain occurred, don't bend, twist, or lift. Also, don't reach above head height.

After a back injury, you should approach sex the way porcupines do: very carefully. It's probably better to avoid vigorous sex for a day or two, because, in case you had not noticed, it often involves repeated impact from and to the lower back and pelvic area. It might sound like a good way to cheer you up and take your mind off your bad back, but it isn't.

In anything you attempt to do, think balance. Even to pick up and drink a glass of water, use both hands. When you're getting dressed, sit on the bed or a chair to get into pants, tights, socks, shoes. In other words, don't do anything standing so that you have to balance on one leg. It may sound silly, but while you're recovering it's important to maintain stability, and any amount of weight or loading on one side will tend to pull your back away from vertical.

HEAT AND COLD

STAY WARM! YOU don't want any other muscles tensing up, and that can easily happen when one group of muscles or ligaments is under strain. Cool air makes blood vessels contract. So put on a sweater and stay out of drafts.

If you just strained your back, especially in an impact injury, and you have obvious signs of inflammation like swelling, heat, or redness, wrap an ice pack in a tea towel or other light fabric so your skin doesn't get "burned" from the cold, and put it on or under your back where it hurts for about twenty minutes. If you don't have an ice pack, you can smash up some ice cubes and put them in a plastic bag. Or better yet, a bag of frozen peas or corn does the trick very nicely, and the little bumps actually feel rather pleasant. The cold will keep the inflammation down, and can reduce pain as well as your recovery time. Apply it for twenty minutes at a time, not more than four times a day for the first day or two. And then you can start the heat.

Heat feels much nicer than cold, and once the inflammation has gone down, it will help restore circulation to the affected muscles and ligaments and speed the healing process. It will also prevent spasms. Don't apply heat if your injury has just happened or if it was due to a blow or a fall. It can increase inflammation, swelling, and pain.

Heat works best when it's moist, as it goes deeper than dry heat. A bath will make you feel a lot better—if the position you would have to be in isn't uncomfortable. But unless you have help getting in and out, it might be easier to take a shower, and it's great to have the stream of water directed right onto the painful spot. You also can't go wrong with a good old hot water bottle. The frumpiest member of the pain-treatment family, the hot water bottle is a cheap, simple method of reducing muscle spasm and pain. You can also get these nifty little "wheat bags" from pharmacies or health food shops that you heat in a microwave and use like any other form of heat therapy.

Like cold, heat should not be applied for more than twenty minutes at a time, or more than a few times a day. Don't use ice or heat in any form if you have a loss of feeling, and if you have any questions, call your practitioner.

MASSAGE

IF YOUR PAIN seems to be of a muscular nature and wasn't caused by sudden impact, you might try using any form of bribery available to get your friend, partner, or any willing relative to give you a massage. You can recognize muscle pain because it's located in muscle tissue next to, but not in, the spine, and you might feel it as a spasm or grabbing pain. We know a woman who got her teenage daughter to give her a massage in exchange for a gift certificate to the local day spa. Remember: everyone has a price. The person doesn't have to be highly trained. Just relatively sensitive, gentle, and of course willing to stop immediately if it makes the pain worse.

If no one is around, you can usually massage yourself for short periods. It's obviously easiest with the neck and lower back, and you should use cream or oil just like the pros. Start gently then get firmer, as long as it doesn't hurt. With hard-to-reach spots, you might want to use any of various massage devices that are available in health food and gift shops. If you have a tennis ball lying around, it can be pressed into service for use in the center of your back on those muscles inside your shoulder blades that are really impossible to massage on your own otherwise. Just place the ball on the floor and lie back on it, rolling over it while it works out your spasm. Sometimes a few well-placed self-inflicted rubs can get you out of immediate trouble until you get to a practitioner, if you end up needing one at all.

RELAX

No MATTER WHAT the cause, most back pain can be lessened somewhat by any number of relaxation techniques. We go into more depth about them in a later chapter as part of a maintenance and prevention plan, but you can certainly find relief in the midst of an attack through meditation, creative visualization, and other techniques designed to help you let go of muscle tension. You can also simply concentrate on relaxing the muscle that's tight. This is easier to do in the early stages of spasm, but sometimes you can get your muscles to relax just by focus and will.

MEDICATE

OF COURSE THERE are drugs, as discussed earlier. Just remember to take only what you really need, and then not for more than a day or two unless told otherwise by your practitioner. With most bad backs, you'll only need something for the first day or two, so don't get into a habit that will be hard to break. Also, don't hesitate to consult your pharmacist about what over-the-counter painkiller would be best for you. They often know as much as doctors about the different properties of each drug they sell. They'll also be able to tell you about a range of creams from tiger balm to anti-inflammatory rubs that can help with superficial muscle tension as well as deeper ligament damage.

At your pharmacy you can also get spinal supports and other gizmos to wear while you recover, but don't get dependent on these and assume they can take the place of well-toned muscles. Another amazing product available at your pharmacy is an herbal plaster, which comes in large patches that you can apply to your back where it hurts. The herbs, including arnica and capsicum, penetrate your skin and give you warm, stimulating sensations that you won't believe are coming from such an innocent-looking square of plastic. And the plaster holds and supports the affected area.

STRETCH/EXERCISE

THERE ARE EXERCISES that can relieve even serious pain, but they are best done after your practitioner or a physical trainer has deemed them appropriate and actually shown you how to do them, and knows that you're doing them safely. If at any time the pain gets worse, stop. It's always a good idea to do exercises and stretching right after a bath or shower, when your muscles are warm and loose. Read the section on stretching (pages 108–110), which goes into more detail about how to stretch. You will see in the following photos that different people have different degrees of flexibility. Remember to do the exercises slowly and gently within your own limits.

Hang-from-a-door

One ridiculously simple decompression exercise is to hang from a door by your hands. You'll want to check first to see that the door will take your weight; if this looks risky, find something else with similar height and stability. If you have an exercise bar placed high in a doorway, that's perfect. If you do use a door, you might want to throw a towel over the top to cushion your hands. Then just grip the top of the door tightly and lift your knees till you can feel your spine lengthening. Do this slowly and gently. You don't have to lift your feet completely off the floor. Just enough to take some of the load off your spine so it can stretch a bit. Take a few long deep breaths, and then take your weight through your legs and feet again, and stand up straight. Do not at any point pull yourself up with your arms. You would be using back muscles, which may already be strained. All you want to do here is reduce the compression of your spine exerted by your own body weight and our old nemesis, gravity.

Knees-to-chest

Another decompression exercise to loosen jammed verte-brae is one where you lie on a mat or soft surface on the floor and bring your knees up as close to your chest as you can, and rock gently back and forth. Try to hold your abdominal muscles in, and don't forget to breathe. It will be easiest to do this if your ankles are crossed. Then try the rocking motion while your knees are spread open and your thighs create a right angle. Roll back and forth and from side to side. Don't worry about how silly you look.

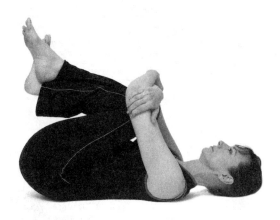

Lumbar stretch

For general stiffness in the lower back, it can feel great just to kneel on the floor and then bend over so your upper body is lying against your knees, your forehead on the floor, and your arms limp on the floor at your sides or stretched out in front of you. Make sure you breathe deeply and low in your diaphragm in this position and you'll get a fabulous stretch through the sacral area and other places you didn't know could stretch!

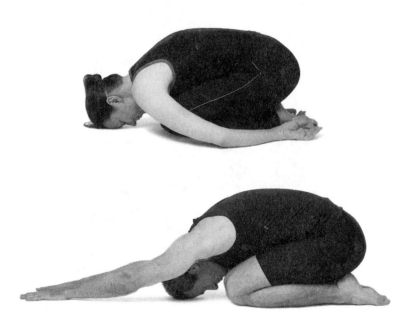

breathe deeply to stretch places you didn't know could stretch!

Thoracic stretch

If you have upper back stiffness that can often come on after too many hours at the computer or sewing machine or any other stationary job, this is a great stretch for you. Get on the floor on all fours, lean over with your right hand extended forward while you're supported on your left elbow. Push your right hand as far as it will go as you breathe deeply and feel the stretch through your upper back and shoulders. Then do the same with your left hand as you're supported on your right elbow. Then extend both hands forward and stretch with your forehead resting on the floor. Pure bliss. Just try to do it on a carpeted floor or a mat to avoid forehead burn.

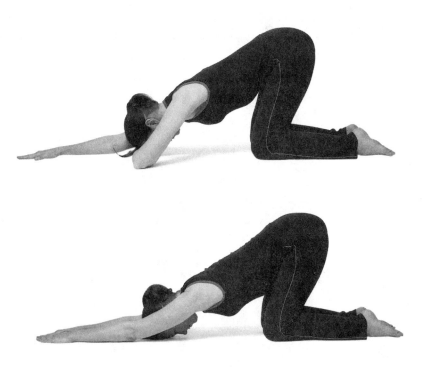

Lumbar squat

Squatting is what smart people do who know that sitting all day isn't good for them. But in your line of work, like chief executive officer or airline pilot, it may not be practical for you to squat on the job. That's why it will be great to do some squatting when you get home. The marvelous thing about a good squat is that you're decompressing the area of the back most prone to damage and injury—the lumbar region. Just hold on to something, like the kitchen sink or a door knob, or do it freestanding if you can, and lower yourself until you're down on your haunches with your feet planted on the floor a comfortable distance apart. Then lean forward a little and breathe deeply, and move around inside the stretch. You can actually feel your pelvis lowering to the floor. Which is a very good thing.

squatting is great for the lumbar region

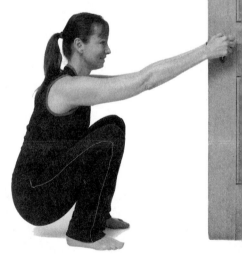

Sitting gluteal stretch

Sometimes pain and stiffness can be referred from a spasm in the gluteal muscles, and by stretching them you can find relief. If it's safe and comfortable for you, sit on the floor with your legs straight in front of you, then bend your right knee and cross it over your left leg so your right foot sits flat on the floor to the left of your left knee. Slowly twist your torso to the right and use your left elbow or hand to hold your right knee toward the left side and stabilize your torso while your right hand rests on the floor behind you with your right arm straight. Breathe gently into this stretch and feel your glute muscles stretching against your hip. Then slowly release and do the other way.

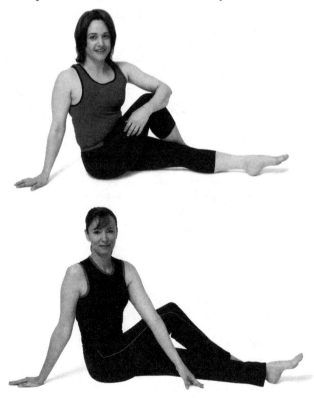

Lying gluteal stretch

Another glute stretch that may be easier depending on what sort of back trouble you have, is one where you lie on your back with your knees bent. Then lift your right leg and rest your ankle on your left thigh near the knee. Reach under your right leg so that your hands grip the outside of your left shin. If this is too hard, hold the back of your thigh. Then gently pull your left leg toward you and that will bring your right leg with it, giving a nice deep stretch to your right gluteal. Release slowly and do your left glute.

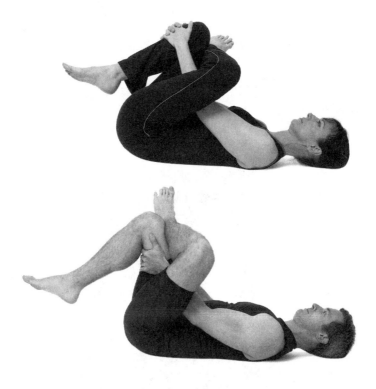

lie down and give your gluteals
a nice deep stretch

Hamstring stretch

Another trick is good for treating some sciatic pain, and is also a great preventative stretch. Lie on your back, then hook a rolled-up towel or belt or scarf around the heel of the foot on the side where you're experiencing pain. Extend your leg in the air, keeping your knee bent, using the towel to guide and steady it. Gently stretch your leg by pulling the towel toward you. If you are able to do the stretch with your leg straight, even better. The goal is to stretch your hamstring muscle and release pressure on the sciatic nerve. You often see runners and other athletes doing a hamstring stretch by sitting on the ground with their legs splayed in front them, and leaning over each leg to get to that area in the back of the thigh. But this position can be bad for people with back trouble as your lower back is not protected, and it can be rough on your neck too. But flat on your back it feels great because you're not doing any bending or compressing. Do it a few times gently, while breathing deeply and holding the stretch comfortably. With certain kinds of sciatica, this can bring instant relief.

a great stretch to release pressure
on the sciatic nerve

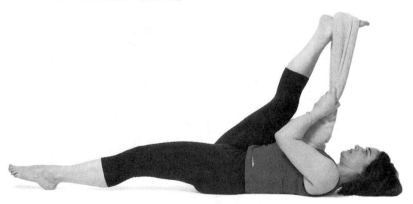

Neck and shoulder stretch

This is a simple little stretch for people who stare at computer monitors for too long. Gently tilt your head to one side as you drop the opposite shoulder using your lat muscles to gently pull it down. Hold for five to ten seconds. Repeat on the other side. Then tilt your head back just until you feel a stretch and hold for another five to ten. Then tilt your head forward slightly for another stretch and hold for five to ten.

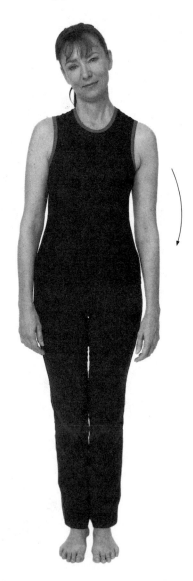

a great stretch for computer users

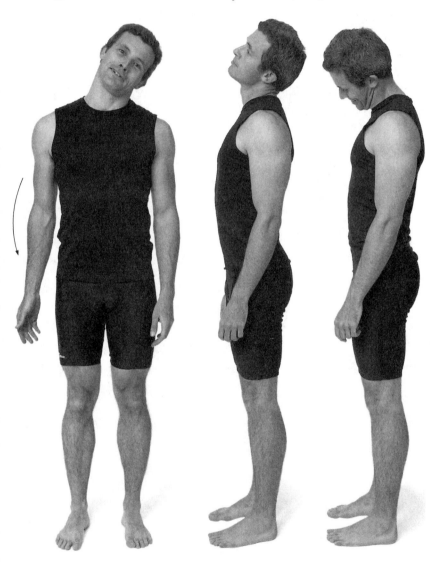

Horizontal twist

No, it's not a '60s dance craze. It's a fantastic stretch for your whole back that puts very little pressure on your discs and can return a lot of spinal mobility to you that may have been lost in strains or injuries. Don't do it if you have a herniated or prolapsed disc. Lie on your back with your arms extended out at the sides with your palms on the floor, then raise your right knee and swing it slowly over your body so it touches the floor on your left side (or as near as you can), while trying to keep your right shoulder and arm as close to the floor as possible. Then breathe. You may hear some clicks and crunches, but don't worry—this should be music to your ears as it signals the release of tight joints. Then slowly do it the other way.

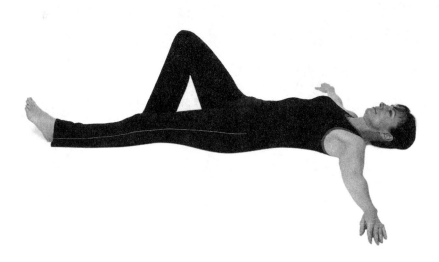

clicks and crunches signal
the release of tight joints

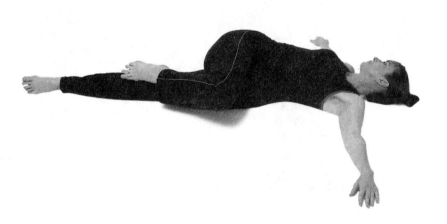

Thoracic stretch

With your hands and arms in a prayer position, rest your hands and elbows against a wall at chest height, then step back to straighten your back and legs, your knees under your hips. Then lower your chest and head below your arms. Some people will get a nice mid-back stretch out of this, but others need to do the bend with their arms extended, hands resting on a windowsill to achieve the same result.

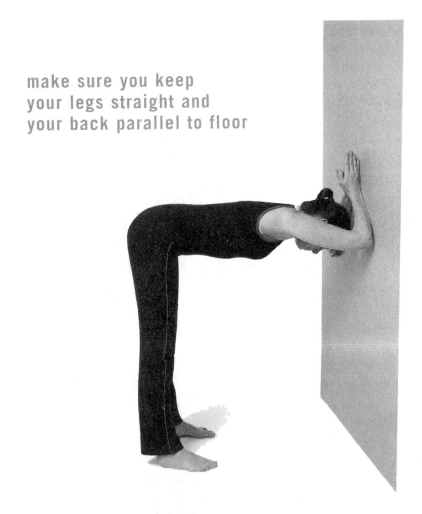

make sure you keep
your legs straight and
your back parallel to floor

Breathing

One of the main reasons that you want to breathe deeply and slowly while you're stretching is to oxygenate your muscles, but there are actually more therapeutic properties to this wonderfully simple thing. When you take a deep breath and fill your lungs you're actually expanding and supporting your back structures from the inside. It's the airbag effect that not only protects your internal structures and frees jammed joints, but also stretches the muscles and ligaments of your back that might be tight from your injury or strain from the inside. And if you want to be really nice to your lower back, you can make sure that you fill your lower lungs and expand your diaphragm first. It's amazing what you can unlock with a few good gulps of air. Slow, deep breathing will also relieve mental tension, which is often one of the guilty parties that put your back out of whack in the first place.

Listen

Above all, listen to your body. Your own instincts are powerful tools. If something doesn't feel right, don't do it. And don't push yourself just because you want to stick to some sort of recovery timetable. Your body, and especially your back, because it has so many different parts that heal at different rates, will let you know when you can start sitting up, riding your bike, moonwalking.

But at the same time, don't hide behind what might feel like instinct but you recognize as fear. After a back strain, it's very easy to be overly wary about reinjuring yourself. Take it slow, stay relaxed, but keep moving, and listen to the messages your body continually sends you.

7 HOW TO MAKE SURE BACK PAIN DOESN'T COME BACK TO HAUNT YOU

Once you've treated your back successfully and are free from pain it's very tempting just to sit back and do exactly what you did before the pain started. That might work for a few days, a few weeks, or even a few months if you're lucky. But don't be a schmuck. If you fall back into the same bad habits, your pain will return. It might start small but it will eventually get bigger and bigger until you're back where you started: in traction and begging for another hit of Demerol.

The secret to keeping your back pain-free is variety. You need to practice a variety of things, from stress management to good posture to exercise. And within your exercise program, once again, variety is the key. Weight training is great, but not if it's the only thing you do. Same goes for running. And lifting cheeseburgers.

What follows is a brief survey of different things you can do to maintain a healthy, happy back. It's not likely that just one of them will do it all. But a couple of them in rotation should do the trick. Once again, it's up to you to discover what works for you. A lot of it is just about what you like doing. Some people like a brisk walk, while for others this is as much fun as watching paint dry. The more social experience of going to the gym inspires some, while for others it's as dull as dishwater.

Of course any exercise routine should only be done after checking with a practitioner you trust. Whether it's your osteopath or your physiotherapist or your orthopedic surgeon, you should check with them before starting something new if back problems have darkened your past. They'll give you some general "dos" and "don'ts," as well as anything to be avoided in your special case.

The other thing to remember when trying a new routine is that pain and/or numbness are signals telling you to stop. Even exercises as user-friendly as yoga, walking, and swimming can lead to problems if you're not doing them right or you've had specific injuries that limit what you can do. We're not talking about the rather pleasant pain that comes after gently pushing your muscles to become stronger by safely increasing their load. We're talking about pain, pins and needles, or numbness triggered by injury or strain. So learn to listen to your body and distinguish the subtle differences in the ways it speaks to you.

Ultimately, everyone is different, and there's a special combination of activities out there that will fit you like a glove. While finding that combination can take some time and effort, the journey can be fun. Don't be afraid to try something that sounds weird or hard or new—and don't be afraid to move on if it's not working or you just don't like it. Remember, there is a solution, and it's your job to find it!

POSTURE

LIKE MOST THINGS about us, the posture we have is a combination of nature and nurture—what we were born with and what we've developed. Sometimes we're born with a condition that makes good posture difficult or impossible, like scoliosis or spina bifida, but most of us are capable of sustaining positions that are good for us. The first thing to realize is that good posture is the most basic ingredient in back maintenance. The second step is knowing what's good.

Strictly speaking, there's no exactly right way to stand or sit. There are only different right ways for different people, depending on their body shape, size, strength, flexibility, and other factors. But we can give you a few pointers.

Remember that the key is balance. This means that when standing, your head, shoulders, hips, knees, and heels should all be in a relatively straight vertical line. You need to find your center and get comfy with it. The weight of your body should fall a little in front of your ankle joints. In any other position, for example with your shoulders rounded forward or your knees locked back, your muscles will have to compensate to keep you stable—in other words, to keep you from tipping over. This will eventually result in overuse in some areas and under-use in others. The long-term effect will be misalignment and undue stress and strain leading to pain. But if you've already had back pain and you've been successfully treated, the trick is now to make sure that bad habits are replaced by good ones, and they start with good posture.

The other key to good posture is that you should be able to maintain a balanced position with your muscles relaxed rather than tensed. If all you're doing is standing or sitting, and you can feel tension in a certain area, those muscles are probably overcompensating for an imbalance or area of weakness somewhere else.

When you move, avoid bending from the waist, unless you can support yourself by holding onto something. Avoid crossing your legs and feet for long periods, especially if you have a history of back problems, as the position de-stabilizes your spine. Cross your legs now and feel what it does to your lower back: it puts everything out of balance and strains the muscles unevenly. Then uncross them and feel the comfort of being in balance.

Often books will tell you that "perfect posture" is when you're standing upright, your weight is balanced evenly, with your feet slightly spread apart, pointed straight ahead. This is fine if you want to look like a nightclub bouncer, but for the rest of us, that pose is not all that realistic. It's fine to shift your weight from side to side every once in a while. Just try not to favor one side more than the other.

It's not good to hold even a great posture for a long time. It's always important to move. Even in our sleep we roll around a good bit, up to fifty times a night being normal. A variety of good postures is what you want to aim for. Like a supermodel. Without the high heels. And that bored look on your face.

If you have difficulty changing your postural habits, some of the exercises and disciplines that follow, including yoga, tai chi, Pilates, Feldenkrais, and Alexander Technique, can be of great help. Not only will they give you more strength and flexibility, they'll put you in touch with your body and how it moves in a way that will change your fundamental postural habits. In short, they'll make good posture automatic and unconscious, rather than something you have to strive for. You may even find that slumping becomes uncomfortable!

In the meantime, just remember that with posture, the important things are relaxation, balance, and stability.

STRESS MANAGEMENT

THERE'S NO SUCH thing as life without stress. Even if it were possible, we wouldn't want to eliminate stress completely. Stress inflames our passions and spices up our often boring days with excitement. Stress gives life an edge.

We need stress to stimulate us to fulfill our goals. For example, don't most of us work better on a deadline? We know that if we didn't have one for this book, it would still be unfinished when people are taking weekend vacations on Mars. Stress helps us organize and prioritize. It guides us in time management and can push us to perform better and for longer. But when stress is excessive, it can lead to problems.

Most people carry their excess stress in the same places day after day. One of the most common spots is across the back of the neck and the tops of the shoulders. Others wear their stress in the lower back. Still others feel it in their digestive systems, some of which can be brought on by pressure on nerves in a tense neck. Why do you think that when you have a massage, these are the areas that get the most attention? What you want to do is get to stress before it gets to you and your back. You need to learn how to manage stress.

The good news is that there are lots of widely practiced methods of stress management, and none of them requires expensive equipment or that you join some strange religion. And the great thing is that once you find the technique that works for you, not only a pain-free back, but general good health and a sense of well-being can be yours.

Creative visualization

Your imagination is like a muscle. It's one of the greatest tools you have, but it's often underused, and if you haven't used it in a while you might think you don't even have an imagination. Well, guess what? Everybody does, and the more you use it, the stronger it will get. A strong imagination is a potent weapon against stress. How? It's called creative visualization.

The profound physical effect of picturing something in your head has been proven in many different scientific tests. For example, it has been demonstrated that if someone merely imagines that he is lifting heavy weights, there is significant muscle activity. Also, people recovering from throat surgery are advised not to read because it's been found that their throats actually work to shape the words on the page. You can prove it yourself if you imagine that your hand is warming itself near an open fire. Imagine the experience intensely, and that hand will actually get warmer. Or think of biting into a lemon and no doubt your mouth will water. There's nothing mystical about this. It's simply a matter of the mind dictating how the body responds.

What all this means is that if you imagine yourself in a safe, peaceful, comfortable place, your body will respond accordingly. For you, it might be in a warm bath in an opulent bathroom. Or having a massage. Or lying on a beach being fanned by Brad Pitt (which might have physical effects other than relaxation). Whatever the image is, it will stimulate subtle muscle movements. Your visualization can actually relax your body, and those muscles that would gradually tighten into painful little knots actually loosen and lengthen. This is a pleasant, simple way to keep stress from getting the better of you.

Meditation

One of the most widely accepted and effective stress management techniques is meditation. If you haven't already enjoyed its benefits, it may be because you associate it with a spiritual movement that isn't up your alley. Or you think you wouldn't do it right. Or you would get bored. Don't let those ideas put you off any longer. Meditation has been proven to lower blood pressure, decrease adrenaline output, improve memory and overall mental dexterity, as well as aid in recovery from illness. It can also lead to all sorts of self-discoveries. There is really nothing quite like it. And it's free!

Don't tell us you don't have the time. Meditation will actually give you more useable time because you'll feel better and think more efficiently. In today's society, we often feel as though our brains are radios with all the stations playing at once. This is mental multitasking taken to a dangerous extreme, and you need to be able to turn the radio off or at least set it to one quiet station every once in a while if you don't want to blow a fuse.

There's simply no way around it: meditation is for everybody and it can help you unwind in less time than it takes to drink a double martini.

So what is meditation?

Put simply, meditation is a state of extreme relaxation achieved through rhythmic breathing and the clearing of the mind. For some people, it occurs naturally when they're working or exercising, especially during something even and rhythmic like running. There are dozens if not hundreds of ways of meditating, with loads of classes, books, audiotapes, and Web sites devoted to various techniques. Like everything, you need to find the way that suits you. When you're starting out, it will help to get some guidance from a teacher or a doctor or a friend. These days, more and more general practitioners, specialists, and counselors suggest that their patients learn to meditate because they know what the physical and psychological benefits can be. Take their advice.

In the meantime, here are the basics.

Get into a position where you feel comfortable and relaxed. Eliminate distractions like people, TV, Kettle Chips. You don't have to sit cross-legged but you can. If you're seated in a chair, make sure that your back is supported and your feet are planted evenly on the floor.

You can close your eyes or keep them open—whatever you're more comfortable with. Then just start breathing slowly and deeply. When you do this, use the lower part of your lungs. This is called diaphragmatic breathing, as your diaphragm rather than your chest expands and contracts as you breathe. Diaphragmatic breathing is better for you all the time, whether you're meditating or not. There are more oxygen-absorbing blood vessels in the lower lungs, and the increased use of the diaphragm better supports your lower back. This also takes pressure off other muscles in the neck and shoulders that tend to overwork.

Breathing is the key to all meditation. Not only will it relax you physically, it will help you empty your mind of unwanted thoughts because you'll be focused on inhaling and exhaling. The extra oxygen from deep breathing stimulates the release of endorphins, hormones that will boost your mood. This is the really fun part.

It can also be useful to have a word or phrase that you repeat with each inhale/exhale sequence. In Eastern meditation, this is called a mantra. The beauty of a mantra is that you get to pick it. It can be anything in the world as long as it's a word or phrase that helps you relax. It might be the word, "calm" or something like "ocean," or "chocolate mud cake"—whatever—each syllable corresponding to the inhale or the exhale. Or it might be just a sound.

You can say your mantra out loud or inside your head. Whatever it is, both the meaning of the word and the image it conjures up should be peaceful and reassuring. Like breathing, a mantra helps you keep your mind off the bills you have to pay, the boss who's giving you grief, or your kids who sometimes demand a lot of your sanity, your time, and your cash.

Invariably, thoughts like these will intrude anyway—but don't fight them.

Just let them in, and then let them go. Keep coming back to your breathing and your mantra.

Some people like to use creative visualization when they meditate. As you breathe deeply (with or without a mantra) you might be able to relax more easily if you imagine a peaceful scene where you feel happy, relaxed, safe. It might be a real place—a childhood bedroom or your favorite holiday spot. Or it could be a place you've made up—a perfect garden of tropical flowers and sweet-smelling fruit with a hammock under a palm tree in which you can relax without a care in the world. Whatever it is, images, rather than the absence of images, might help you empty your head of worries.

Guided meditation and visualization audiotapes can be great at giving you something to focus on as your mind and body relaxes, and might be particularly helpful for those of you who don't feel confident about getting started on your own.

One of the great things about meditation is that you don't have to spend an hour or half an hour or even fifteen minutes doing it. Obviously a daily dose of at least twenty minutes will help you enormously, but you can calm yourself and manage stress by breathing and clearing your mind any time, anywhere, if you feel it creeping up on you.

For example, if you have to make a speech—an event that can bring on massive stress—you can do some deep breathing and recite your mantra in your head as you walk up to the podium. Or in an elevator on your way to a job interview; or just before you begin a test; or on the way to your wedding. Whatever stresses you out.

By freeing your mind and body—even for a few seconds—from the sources of stress, you can lose the tension that manifests itself as muscle tightness among other things. This way, you can prevent back pain from taking hold. Put out that flame while it's just on the head of a match and it won't set fire to the whole forest.

Aromatherapy

We all know how powerful scents are. A smell can evoke a memory with astounding accuracy. Places, people, and the mood we were in when we last encountered them can be brought back in amazing detail when triggered by a certain fragrance. But this usually happens accidentally. The good news is that we can trigger positive thoughts and emotions on purpose, through the use of essential oils.

The soothing, healing properties of plant extracts have been known since the ancient Egyptians used them, but they've enjoyed a renaissance in the last quarter century. Particularly as a way to manage stress, aromatherapy is simple, inexpensive, and pleasurable.

Essential oils are derived from various plants at maturity for the greatest potency. They can then be used in several ways—burned, in the bath, inhaled directly, or massaged into the skin.

For burning, just add the oil of your choice to an oil burner that uses the heat from a candle below the suspended oil bowl. The fragrance will permeate the room in a pleasant but subtle way and can help you keep your cool while you're working, relaxing, meditating, or helping with the kids' algebra.

Adding a few drops to your bath is especially good for stress-related back pain, because the warm water will help your muscles relax while the aroma settles your mind.

Essential oils added to a neutral massage oil and massaged into your skin can also be a fantastic way to unload stress and turn a rotten day into a magnificent evening.

You can also add the oil to warm water in a bowl, cover your head, and inhale the vapors, or just add a few drops to a handkerchief and sniff it when you need to chill out.

Here are some of the essential oils that are particularly good at keeping stress at bay:

Bergamot	emotionally uplifting, also great for reducing anxiety
Chamomile	calms, relaxes, soothes
Clary sage	uplifting to the point of euphoria, can help fight off mild depression
Frankincense	relaxing, protective; good for meditation
Jasmine	upbeat; induces a sense of well-being
Lavender	really great for stress relief and associated conditions, like sleeplessness
Marjoram	sedative, calming
Neroli	sedative, antidepressant
Peppermint	soothes while it refreshes
Rose	emotionally comforting
Sandalwood	excellent for beating mental stress
Ylang-ylang	euphoric; superb at quelling tension and anger

There are many more essential oils that you can learn about through books or from your local health food store. Don't use them during pregnancy without the advice of a professional, as there are a few that can potentially cause miscarriage. As with everything else, what will work best for you is partly a matter of personal taste. So experiment. There will probably be one or two scents that you find work like a charm.

Buteyko breathing

Also known as eucapnic breathing, the Buteyko breathing technique was developed by a Russian doctor of the same name, and is best known for the benefits it brings asthmatics. It also has been shown to lead to a stronger immune system, more energy-efficient metabolism, and a dramatic fall in stress levels.

Most of us think of carbon dioxide (CO_2) as merely the waste gas we emit when we exhale, but it also regulates many of our bodies' systems. CO_2 is actually a more important stimulator to the respiratory center in our brain than oxygen. The way to maintain healthy levels of CO_2 is through the way we breathe. Inefficient breathing can lead to hyperventilation, asthma, and general ill health.

Many of us have had the nasty experience of hyperventilating during an anxiety or panic attack—when stress levels are off the charts. We get rid of too much CO_2 and can't "catch" our breath. We sweat, our hearts race, we might even notice palpitations. With Buteyko, or eucapnic breathing (eucapnic means "normalizing CO_2"), not only is this condition avoided, but we actually reduce our stress levels and induce a feeling of calm. Stress arouses our nervous systems. Buteyko breathing actually reduces stimulation to the nervous system.

The technique should be learned from a certified Buteyko or eucapnic practitioner, but only after consulting your doctor, especially if you have any respiratory or cardiac conditions.

To give you an idea of the method, it works like this:

Exhale completely. Then exhale a bit more until your abdomen is pulling back against your spine. Hold like that without inhaling for as long as you comfortably can (eventually up to half a minute.) Then slowly and evenly inhale. Breathe the way you would normally for a few cycles, then start again.

You will learn from your practitioner that this method is not to be used only when you are in the middle of a stressful episode, but on a daily basis. It will help to regulate your CO_2 levels and keep anxiety, as well as other health problems, at bay.

Common sense solutions

At the risk of stating the obvious, there are a lot of basic things you can do to manage your stress levels, but sometimes under the weight of all that blinding pressure, you forget what they are. By way of refreshing your memory:

◆ Talk to your friends. Keeping your problems bottled up inside is the surest way of getting the kind of tension that will manifest itself in your muscles. The very act of sharing these problems with a friend over a cup of coffee or a glass of vino somehow helps to spread the load. Even if you don't get any useful advice, you'll realize that everybody has problems, and sometimes that's enough to bring you back from the brink of stress-burnout.

◆ Go for a walk. We're not talking "power walking" or any form of muscle-toning or cardiovascular exercise. We just mean getting out the door and moving through some alternate scenery to the one that's giving you grief. It doesn't have to be a pretty park or a majestic forest. Sometimes just getting out of the house or office and putting a little physical distance between you and the source of your stress can help. It helps you to see that however awful they seem, your problems probably don't amount to a hill of beans in this crazy world.

Unless you're the president. In which case, get your ylang-ylang out.

◆ Don't get obsessed with the news. We're not suggesting you adopt a head-in-the-sand attitude, but you should not fixate on a repetitive overabundance of media-disseminated nasty rumors and tragic information. Whether it's on the way to work in the morning or when you get home at night, many of us tune into talk radio or broadcast news, and in our vulnerable state —commuting—we take the crises of the world (wars, famine, floods, serial killers, TV ratings) on our shoulders. Which consequently sag (literally!) and cause back fatigue. Try a talking book (if you're in your car or on public transport) or read a book, or play with your kids if you're at home. As the poet Robert Frost said when asked why he didn't read newspapers,

"I figure if something really important happens, my friends will tell me about it."

◆ Drink moderately. Now, moderately doesn't mean a mere six-pack of beer or only a couple of bottles of wine. Moderately means about two to three standard drinks per day for men, and around half that or less for women. Obviously this depends on the individual and it's your job to find out what's enough for you. As we all know, even a little booze doesn't agree with some people at all. But for the rest of you, a small amount can be beneficial. Recent studies into longevity and mental as well as physical health have concluded that moderate drinking actually appears to be better for you than not drinking at all. This is partly to do with the chemical effects of alcohol, particularly red and white wine, but mostly it's the relaxing/uplifting effects. How civilized to come home from work to a martini or a glass of red. Tasty, too. Just don't forget that excessive drinking has the reverse effect and is a terrible depressant.

- Drink lots of water. Stress dehydrates us, so you want to minimize this effect.
- Get a life. You should work to live, not live to work. Having interests like hobbies, classes, community service, and of course a broad social life helps put your work stresses as well as relationship stresses into perspective, usually making them seem more manageable.
- Remember the simple pleasures and make time for them in your busy schedule. Good food, good sex, and a good night's sleep are all things that sometimes get lost in the shuffle when we're trying to squeeze twenty-eight hours into twenty-four. Put them back on the top of your priorities list and you'll be a less stressed-out person. More popular, too.
- Then there's exercise. Any form of physical exercise that you can do safely will help you manage stress. You'll feel better, breathe easier, and think more clearly and calmly if you get regular exercise at least three or four times a week. In the sections following, we give an overview of exercises that will cater to a huge variety of tastes. With a little patience and a sense of adventure, you'll find at least one or two that are meant for you.

Medication

For years, a lot of people with long term stress management problems took different kinds of medication—often tranquilizers, such as valium—to keep from going off the deep end. There are problems, however, with taking medication for long periods, and most of us are now aware of them: a variety of psychological and physical side effect including dependency.

Before you resort to prescription medication to control your stress levels, try other solutions, like the ones mentioned in this book or others that safely help you cope with life's little challenges, like marriage and employment. Don't confuse the effects of stress with depression or other psychological conditions. Prozac isn't going to get rid of stress for you, although it may seem to be the easy way out. The better way out may seem to take more effort but it will be much more fun in the long run.

STRETCHING

WHEN YOU WAKE up in the morning, before you get out of bed, take a minute to stretch gently. Your back, arms, legs, neck—just a few mild extensions. You'll be less stiff and feel better right away. But don't stop there.

Stretching is one of the best things you can do for the health of your back. The goal of stretching is to elongate your muscles, tendons, and other soft tissue so that your joints can move more freely. Stretching moves the joints away from patterns they can get stuck in, and releases the tension held in the muscles and ligaments. This means you can move more efficiently—and without pain.

After those little wake-up stretches you can do in bed, the best time to stretch is after you've had a shower or bath. The warm water will have relaxed your muscles, making them receptive to a good extension. Before you get dressed, lie down on a carpeted floor or a mat and do the basic stretches we described in the Do-It-Yourself section. They're great preventative exercises, so if you want to keep back trouble from returning, keep them up. They'll undo tightness or knotting that might have occurred in your muscles overnight, and it means that you're starting your day in optimum condition. A few nice stretches can make those long hours at a desk or behind a wheel or on your feet much more comfortable.

Of course there are lots of stretching classes and books, and as with every other kind of workout, check with your practitioner before you take the plunge.

As you do each stretch, think about it. Picture the muscles relaxing, lengthening. Remember always to use your mind in conjunction with your body—and keep breathing steadily throughout. You need to keep the oxygen flowing to your muscles so they can handle the stretch.

Don't rush it. Let your muscles elongate in their own good time. And don't bounce when you're stretching. We see this all the time, and it's not doing your body any favors. You can risk tearing muscles, tendons, and tissues, and even bring on serious injury.

One of the most common mistakes people make is to unconsciously tense muscles other than the ones they're stretching. For instance, when people stretch their calf muscles, they often tense their neck and shoulders, which is not a good idea. So try to consciously relax your other muscles. Or put your body in a position so that other muscles don't come into play. This is different from the practice in yoga where there is intentional tensing of muscles away from the one you're stretching. For example, in a hamstring stretch, you might purposely contract your quadriceps (front thigh muscles), which actually causes greater relaxation in the hamstring.

Stretch to where it's within easy and comfortable range, and then gently stretch a little further. Do this by relaxing the muscle as you breathe out, and then follow the exhale with a gently applied further stretch. Never stretch to where you feel pain. After a while, you'll get to know your body, and will be able to feel just how far to go. But always be on the safe side. Even movement within an easy range will increase oxygen to the area. Remember that there is no right range; it's whatever distance gives you a good, safe stretch.

Most people don't hold a stretch long enough. Don't just go into your stretch, get there, and get out. Maintain the point of stretch comfortably while you breathe for at least fifteen seconds, and longer for greater benefits. Then gently and progressively release the stretch, making sure the rest of your body moves easily, without jerks or pulls.

Make sure you stretch after a workout. As you exercise, your muscle cells generate heat, increasing flexibility, but as they cool, they shorten. That's why even with a work-out as innocuous as walking, you should do some basic stretches to avoid injury and strain. You should also stretch after you've been in one position for a long time. You need to reoxygenate those muscles to maintain flexibility and stability.

Some recent studies suggest that stretching before you exercise is unnecessary. But if you feel excessive stiffness in a specific area, try warming it up before you put it to work with a gentle stretch. In any case, if you don't stretch, you need to do some sort of warmup before exercise.

The more you get to know your body and where it likes to be stretched, you can adapt the stretches described here or other stretches to suit your needs. As always, it's a good idea to check with your trainer or back-care practitioner to make sure your variation is safe. But usually your body will tell you pretty quickly whether or not you're doing the right thing.

BASIC BACK EXERCISES

SOME FUNDAMENTAL TRUTHS about exercise:

+ If you exercise, you'll recover from back pain more quickly and are more likely to remain pain-free in the future.
+ Exercise is addictive. Embrace your addiction.
+ Rushing through your exercises is bad.
+ It's good to exercise at least three or four times a week. If you exercise more often, make sure you take one day off a week.
+ Exercise that causes pain is bad.

- There's no right time of the day to exercise. Some people get the most out of a morning workout, while others like it after work. It's your call.
- Exercise aids digestion and reduces constipation.
- Cross-training is good. As with everything else, variety is not only more fun and less boring, but it's better for you.
- Stretching before you exercise is good, but stretching after you workout is really essential.
- It's wise to consult with your back-care practitioner before you start an exercise program. Some exercises are great for some backs and bad for others, depending on your history. Don't be too gung ho and rush into something that could hurt you.
- You're less likely to view exercise as work if you do it with a friend or partner or even the kids.
- Exercising is fun. So enjoy yourself!

In addition to the stretches already described, there are some basic strengthening exercises that are essential in maintaining a healthy and pain-free back. Obviously there are a lot of other exercises that focus on different parts of your body, but these are designed particularly for your back and abdominal muscles and should be regularly included in your exercise program.

With the ones that you do on the floor, it's best to lie on a thin padded exercise mat, or at least a towel or two on top of carpeting.

Pelvic tilt

Lie on your back, knees bent, feet flat on the floor, arms at sides. In this neutral position your lower back will be slightly raised from the floor. Now, rotate your pelvis so your lower back presses into the floor by engaging your abdominal muscles. Imagine pushing with your bellybutton into the floor. Hold for five seconds. Keep breathing. Relax. Repeat five to ten times.

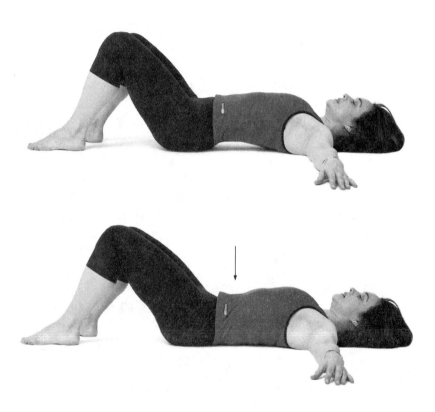

a great, easy exercise
for your back and tummy

Butt rise

Lie on your back, knees bent, feet flat on the floor, arms at your sides. Slowly raise your butt in the air by engaging your abdominal, gluteal, and leg muscles and rolling upward. Hold for three to ten seconds.

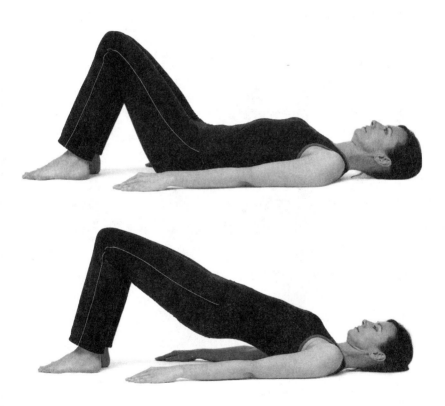

exercise your tummy, glutes, and legs while you improve lower back posture

Leg rotation

Lie on your back, knees bent, feet flat on floor, arms extended out. Bring your knees towards your chest, then lower them slowly to one side as far as is comfortable, turning your head in the opposite direction. Use your abdominal muscles to stabilize, and keep that bellybutton sucked in. Hold for a few seconds then slowly bring both knees up and over to the opposite side in the same way. Repeat five to ten times.

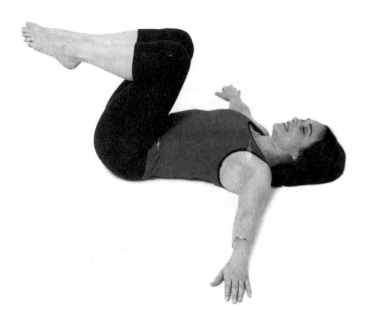

excellent for the abdominal muscles

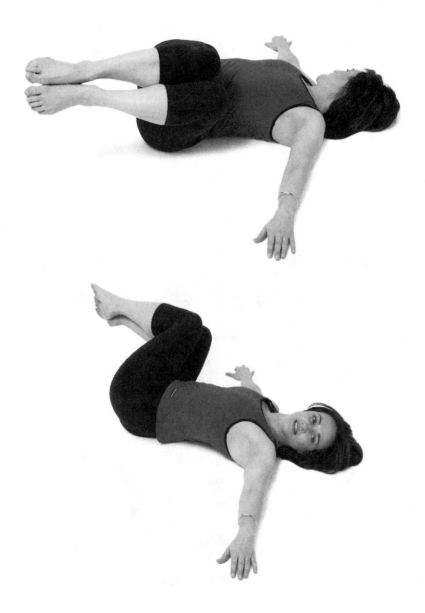

Coffee table

Kneel on all fours and engage your abdominals so your bellybutton is pulled back toward your spine. Keep your back straight and your pelvis stable as you slowly raise your right leg to a horizontal position. Hold for three to five seconds then bend your knee, raise and hold, then lower. Do the same with the left side. Make sure your trunk stays flat, top and bottom, like a coffee table. Repeat five to ten times.

great for your lower back, abdominals, and glutes

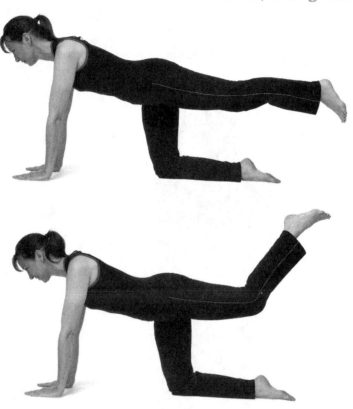

Cobra

Lie face down with your legs straight and arms bent with your hands on the floor under your shoulders. Straighten your arms as far as you can and push your torso up to vertical, keeping your pelvis as close to the floor as possible. Breathe deeply and let your spine drop down as you hold the position. Don't hunch your shoulders and neck. Reverse the process to lie down. Repeat.

This exercise feels remarkably good as it stretches your abdominals and the front of your discs and other soft tissues in the spine. Make sure to check with your practitioner about this one because in some cases it may not be recommended.

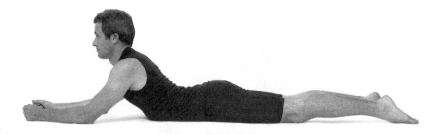

stretch your abdominals and breathe deeply

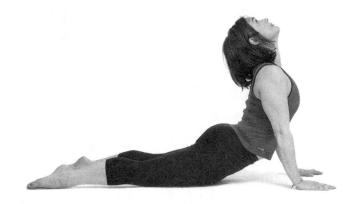

Diagonal reach

Lie on your back, knees bent, feet flat on floor, arms at your sides. With your abdominal muscles engaged, belly-button pulling inward, lift your torso on the left side and reach with your left arm toward the right side of your right knee. Then lie back, and do it to the left side with your right arm. Repeat five to ten times.

great for your abdominals
and your upper back

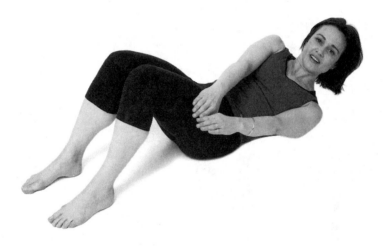

While doing all these exercises, don't forget to breathe. Some people have the mistaken impression that you have to exhale as you pull your abdominal muscles in, but you should be able to take deep diaphragmatic breaths while your bellybutton is pulling into your spine. The more you breathe with these muscles engaged, the sooner it will become a subconscious, automatic behavior, and you'll be protecting and supporting your back without even thinking about it.

This is a basic beginner's drill. Your practitioner will be able to recommend more exercises that you can add that are tailored to your needs and abilities.

INVERSION DEVICES

THERE ARE A number of apparatus designed to decompress your spine with you upside down. Years ago, inversion boots were popular. They were boots that you could hook onto a horizontal rod so you could hang there and let your spine elongate with gravity on your side. But these were tricky to use, and a few people fell out of them, landing on their heads.

Since then various swings and inversion harnesses have been developed that work on the same principle, but are safer because you're actually strapped into a frame that you get into while it's vertical, then it swings around 180 degrees until you're hanging like a bat. Some gyms and even amusement parks have these, and they can feel great and are lots of fun as a novelty if nothing else.

YOGA

YOGA IS BY far one of the nicest things you can do for your back because it's such a holistic exercise, uniting body, mind, and spirit through postures and breathing. In fact the word *yoga* means "union." Because it tones, strengthens, and stretches while also helping you manage stress, it's a wonderfully integrated workout. And you don't have to be an Olympic athlete to do it.

The basic principles of yoga were developed around five thousand years ago in India and haven't fundamentally changed since. Hatha yoga is the physical, as opposed to the spiritual, side of yoga, and it involves doing a range of poses along with controlled breathing. Which is not to say that it isn't spiritual.

In Hindu, prana is the essential life force in all things. Yoga is about keeping our pranic energy balanced so we stay healthy and happy. According to yogic tradition, pranic energy flows through different pathways or channels in the body, much like acupuncture meridians. There are three main channels: one that runs up and down the spine, and two on either side that intersect several times and connect in the forehead. In hatha yoga, you'll learn to maximize the flow of energy along these channels.

There are nearly 200 hatha yoga postures, with hundreds of variations that come with inspiring names like "the hero" and "the warrior." Their primary goal is to make the spine supple, the muscles toned, and to enhance circulation throughout your organs, tissues, and glands. Through stretching and alignment, the poses make your body more balanced and flexible, which is essential in maintaining a pain-free back.

Like all forms of exercise, you need to check with your practitioner to make sure yoga is safe for you. In most cases, he or she will be thrilled that you're doing yoga as it addresses some of the most common, basic back problems.

When you're starting out, it's best to be part of a yoga class. Coordinating the stretches, poses, and breathing can be tricky at first so it's best to be guided by a teacher. In selecting what class is right for you, it's useful to understand two of the main types of yoga, Iyengar and Ashtanga.

Iyengar is named for its originator, an Indian yogi (yoga master) whose aim it was to bring every cell of the body to life. In Iyengar yoga, you hold the poses for a long time in order to bring your bones, muscle, and tissue into alignment, or balance. It's a static, exact, focused exercise.

Taking a very different approach, but with the same goals, Ashtanga yoga involves continuous movement and breathing during which you can really work up a sweat. This is Madonna's exercise of choice and you don't hear her complaining about her back. There are different sets of poses in Ashtanga yoga that you learn in a particular sequence, but many people don't move beyond the first set. Don't worry. It's still an amazing workout.

In all hatha yoga, because of the huge range of poses, you'll discover muscles you didn't know you had. Even if you get a little sore, you'll feel the benefits very quickly. Because of the breathing techniques used, your head will be clearer and you'll be less tired. Unlike with some activities, you'll feel better, lighter, and more energized immediately.

The latest trend in yoga is figuratively and literally hot. It is called Bikram yoga, and it's practiced in a room heated to 98.6°F! The theory is that the heat loosens your muscles for deeper stretching, and at the same time you can sweat out all those toxins that have built up in your blood and organs since your last yoga class. And in these classes people do sweat buckets. They also exercise their circulatory system more vigorously than with conventional yoga. Just don't wear something that turns see-through when it gets wet. Because it's a fairly new way to practice yoga, and we can imagine a few risks with this rather extreme form of physical multitasking, we suggest you consider it cautiously.

Once again, which type of yoga you decide to do depends on your own needs, tastes, and the advice of your health professional. There are also some conditions other than your back that you need to consider before trying yoga. One of them is pregnancy. Because of the deep stretching and breathing in sometimes extreme positions, yoga works a lot on your internal organs, and it can have profound effects. So it's not recommended in the first three months, but many schools of yoga give prenatal classes. You also might not want to do yoga at the start of your period—and certainly avoid those upside-down postures. You'll also discover that it's more pleasant to practice yoga on an empty stomach.

If you're interested in yoga, it's worth doing some reading about it because the physical aspect is only a part of the total discipline. The spiritual side may ultimately be as much help for your back problems as the exercises.

TAI CHI AND CHI GUNG

MOST OF US have a vague idea of what tai chi is from seeing people practicing this ancient form of martial arts early morning in the park. They often have their arms raised and move slowly, shifting their weight from one side to the other. Because we're used to rushing through our lives and our exercises, this form of movement might strike us as silly. But trust us, it's anything but.

Tai chi, or tai chi chuan, is one of the oldest of the Chinese martial arts. It was originally designed to slow down martial arts to make them more graceful in a presentation to a visiting king. It later became part of the Taoist "dao" or way, leading to harmony with nature and one's fellow human beings. *Tai chi* means "supreme ultimate" or "great breath," and *chuan* means "fist." Therefore, *tai chi chuan* is "supreme ultimate fist." Fairly pugilistic for something so harmonious!

As in yoga, controlled breathing is basic to the practice of tai chi, and like yoga it is also a very good, gentle exercise for your back as well as your brain, as its goal is to achieve strength through balance, both physical and mental.

Tai chi consists of a series of slow, fluid, connected movements designed to reduce tension, slow down your breathing, and clear your head. While it doesn't have the same obvious muscle-toning and skeletal-aligning benefits as yoga, it works in subtle ways, in smaller increments. It's remarkable how much more aware of your posture you become when you need to move slowly and be sensitive to tiny shifts in your muscles and skeleton to maintain balance.

The slow, deep breathing in tai chi also helps your back because it focuses your energy on a point just below the navel called the dantian or "cinnabar field." When your energy is located at this point, you tend to stay balanced by relying on your abdominal and back muscles to support your spine. The theory is also that this centralized energy can be released in either a gradual way or in a sudden explosion.

It's important that you learn tai chi from a teacher, as the coordination of movement and breathing is so subtle, and the tiny nuances are hard to judge for yourself. As with all exercises, you should check with your practitioner first, but generally, tai chi is so gentle that it won't do you any harm. It's particularly beneficial to older people, or those recovering from illness or surgery, as the exercises are never strenuous.

Closely associated with tai chi, chi gung, or qi gong, was refined around six thousand years ago in northern China, and like other Chinese martial arts, is a discipline that integrates mind, body, and spirit. It has been said that if tai chi is like the body of a car, then chi gung is like the engine. Through a series of low-impact exercises, chi gung focuses on the coordination of meridians to aid the energy flow to our internal organs and the spine. Controlled breathing and stretching used in the exercises can be enormously beneficial to back pain sufferers, and other side effects include increased mental and physical sharpness and strength. They should be teaching these techniques in primary schools along with reading and math.

PILATES

WE ONCE HEARD a Pilates instructor describe the program as "yoga with weights." While this description is somewhat simplistic, it gives you some idea of what the exercises are about.

Essentially, Pilates (puh-lah-teez) uses breath control combined with stretching and strengthening exercises (some with weights as well as other specially designed equipment) in a unique format developed by Joseph Pilates.

Born in Germany in 1880, then moving to England and eventually America, Pilates was chronically ill as a child. Consequently, as an adult, he studied a variety of disciplines including Zen meditation and yoga, as well as Greek and Roman physical regimens, all of which he drew on in developing his exercise program.

The great thing about Pilates for people with back trouble is that it's designed not only for general fitness but for injury recovery and rehabilitation. That's why it's so popular with dancers and athletes. The exercises focus on small, intrinsic muscles rather than large, extrinsic ones. The goals are abdominal strength—instructors call the abdomen our second spine—spinal flexibility, and body control through physical toning and mental focus.

One of the key aspects is that all of this is achieved through quality rather than quantity of movements. Your trainer will supervise you through many different exercises, each repeated in low numbers. This prevents bulk and also keeps you from getting bored! But the point is to concentrate on each incremental movement and coordinate it precisely with your breathing, rather than mindlessly repeat it over and over.

This technique will fortify and tone muscles, open the joints, release tension, and improve posture, flexibility, and balance. You will get a more streamlined body shape—in fact, a "dancer's body," even if you have two left feet—and increased efficiency and fluidity of movement. All of this through exercises that make you more aware of your body as a single, integrated entity.

Some of the equipment is similar to what you would find in an ordinary gym, but much of it is different. Instead of static weights, springs are used, to strengthen as they stretch. A centerpiece of the Pilates studio is the universal reformer, an apparatus that uses your own body weight as well as springs to tone and lengthen your muscles. In one exercise, you get to lie flat on your back with your feet in some stirrups attached to springs as you extend your legs in the air and make froglike movements!

The problem with a lot of gym work is that it's based on isolating muscles and working each area of the body as a separate element rather than treating it as a whole. This often means that certain areas of the body are neglected, or simply not trained to work in concert with the rest. Pilates, especially through a machine like the universal reformer, does the opposite.

Your instructor is always there to keep an eye on your technique. For example, he or she will watch what you're doing with your abdominal muscles as you use hand weights. Or you'll be made aware of your neck wobbling as you work your legs. And you'll always get busted if you forget to breathe.

As always, you should check with your back-care practitioner before doing Pilates, but in most cases you'll be encouraged to enjoy its immense benefits, which include better endurance and strength without increased strain on the lungs and heart. And best of all, your back will be protected while it's being strengthened. Because you're closely guided and supervised by an instructor through your workout, the risk of injury is minimal.

Of course this also means that Pilates isn't cheap. The special equipment at a Pilates studio and the one-on-one instruction means that it's a pretty pricey way to get fit. On the other hand, many Pilates devotees say they can't afford not to do it. The good news is that with increasing popularity, prices in some studios are coming down.

There are also books and videos that will help you do the exercises at home, even if you don't have all the equipment. What a lot of people don't know is that Pilates developed his system first as a series of exercises to be done on a mat on the floor only. The machinery came later. So although it's best to start out with individual supervision, you can do the workout on your own with nothing more than enough space on a floor to stretch out straight. If you do Pilates matwork correctly, you'll discover that your body is the only tool you need to become fit.

Many find that a good way to do Pilates is to go to a studio and get the individual training for a few months while you're learning, then follow up with your own home routine. You can go back for supervised sessions as often as you like, depending on your needs, tastes, and bank balance. Like everything else, you need to come up with a personalized formula that works for you and your back.

ALEXANDER TECHNIQUE

FREDERICK MATTHIAS ALEXANDER (1869–1955) was an actor from Australia who had chronic laryngitis while performing. When no doctor was able to cure him, he started looking at himself in a mirror and watching what he did when he performed. He realized that when he recited his lines, he had the habit of pulling his head back and depressing his larynx. He also figured out that his bad habits involved more than his head and neck. His whole body was involved. Having made the discovery that habitual misuse of the whole body leads to sickness and pain in specific areas, he then developed a technique to retrain the body through simple exercises. What a guy.

The aim of the Alexander Technique is to reduce pain, increase mobility, and provide long-term relief by changing habits you've probably had for decades. Often these habits seem to be the comfortable way of doing things, like slumping in a chair, but they can actually lead to chronic or recurring back pain. What you'll eventually learn through the technique is how to sit upright without strain, head up, spine lengthened, hips balanced. It will give you much greater awareness of how you use your body, and empower you by giving you the means to relieve and prevent your back problems without running to a practitioner three times a week.

Like any other exercise or physical technique, it's best to learn Alexander from a trained professional. Later on you can go it alone, but you'll get it right faster when you start out under the guidance of an expert.

The first phase involves observation of how you do basic things like walking, standing, lifting, sitting. Your teacher will help you see that some of your habitual movements are at the root of your problems. At this point, the teacher will use his or her hands to guide you in a new way of moving. The guidance is gentle and subtle. Initial focus is usually on the head and neck, where so much tension and bad posture create problems in the rest of the body. You'll learn how to let neck and shoulder tension go by embracing what Alexander called the "primary control": the tendency of the spine to lengthen in motion.

Through this process, you'll realize that the way you normally do things often involves unnecessary twists, tensions, pushes, and pulls. The new, better way will feel weird at first because your bones, ligaments, and muscles are used to going another way. This is one of the reasons that it's a good idea to get your directions from a teacher who can watch you instead of trying to learn the technique from a book. What may feel wrong to you might actually be exactly right, and vice versa. Eventually, of course, the new way will feel right, and you'll have retrained your mind and body to function more efficiently, which means without pain.

Most Alexander teachers will also have you lying down in a semisupine position (this means lying on your back on a firm surface with your head supported by a firm, flat mat and your knees up or supported by a chair) for some very basic retraining. Sometimes just lying like this for fifteen minutes or so can relieve symptoms and also help you adjust the fundamental ways you use your body. Your teacher's specific instructions will depend on your particular problems.

Part of the empowering aspect of the technique is in simply returning the element of choice into your behavior. Instead of acting or reacting automatically, you can choose to move a better way. Ironically, after a lot of practice, this will become more and more effortless and you don't have to consciously choose. It will just happen.

Because it's relatively easy and noninvasive, the Alexander Technique has become very popular worldwide, and works especially well along with whatever other treatments you're getting. In fact, many physiotherapists, osteopaths, and chiropractors use basic principles developed by Alexander in their recommendations to patients, such as the idea that you should feel like you're suspended by a string pulling upward from the crown of your head to improve your posture. Like yoga or tai chi or Pilates or any other method of maintaining a pain-free back, Alexander is all about lightness and balance!

FELDENKRAIS

HAVING SOME SIMILARITIES to both Alexander Technique and Pilates, Feldenkrais is a method of exercising and retraining your body and mind to work more efficiently. And when you work efficiently, you can avoid pain.

The method was developed by Dr. Moshe Feldenkrais, who was born in Russia in 1904 and later emigrated to France and then England. An extraordinary man, he was a physicist, a linguist, and the first European to get a black belt in Judo. He also worked on the development of sonar and radar. Talk about variety. He also found time to create one of the most sophisticated fitness techniques there is.

After a serious knee injury he sustained while playing soccer, he combined his understanding of Judo, physics, and biomechanics with newly acquired knowledge of Alexander Technique and neuromuscular physiology to create a method of reprogramming the motor cortex in the brain to change the way we move. Sounds complicated, but the application is deceptively simple. Luckily, Feldenkrais figured out the hard part.

The basis for his approach was the same as Alexander's —that as we grow, we form bad postural and movement habits that result in limited use of our bodies, and of course back pain. There are two stages of the technique, both of which are taught by someone trained in the discipline.

In the first stage, the instructor talks you through a carefully structured sequence of movements while you're either sitting, lying, or standing. This can be done individually or in a group. The idea is that you become aware of how you move as you go through very slow and simple exercises, such as turning your head from side to side as you lie flat on the floor. It's amazing how much you can learn about where your problems are from this.

Like in Pilates, the focus is on the quality of your movements rather than the speed or number of them. Depending on your particular needs, you may be verbally guided through the stages a child goes through in his or her early years, including crawling and walking. What you're doing is unlearning the faulty developmental sequence that led to your present bad habits. Once you've unlearned, you can relearn.

In the second stage, you will do what is called Functional Integration. This is a rather dull way of describing what happens when your instructor uses his or her hands to guide your movements so you get them right. Once again, the theory is that your new, graceful, flowing movements will replace your old, clunky movements, which had been stored in your brain.

As with your first stage, this happens while you're sitting, standing, or lying, and is thoroughly pleasant. You just hang out while your brain passively absorbs the new patterns. Then you do the same movements on your own, and the more you do them the right way, the quicker the brain will respond and make the good movement automatic.

Feldenkrais is great for increasing your body awareness by reinforcing the link between what you think and what you do. In this sense, it's also very empowering, and demonstrates that you have the ability to change your ways, solve your problems, and not let back pain interfere with your life.

Where Pilates is a favorite of dancers, Feldenkrais has often been practiced by musicians, whose habitual static postures and sometimes awkward movement can lead to terrible pain. The wonderful thing about Feldenkrais is that once you've learned the basic technique, you don't have to keep going back, and there's absolutely no special equipment or technology involved. Musical virtuoso concert violinist Yehudi Menuhin loves the exercises because they're so ingenious and yet so simple. That's partly how he makes what he does look effortless.

Feldenkrais, like most of the methods already mentioned, is available in many areas through local schools and colleges, which make them very accessible and much more affordable than they used to be. So, have you run out of excuses yet?

WALKING

GUESS WHAT ALBERT Einstein and Abe Lincoln had in common other than a colorful approach to facial hair? That's right, they were walkers. Even if you're not as smart as they were, or particularly fit, or thin, or young, you can walk, and thus experience one of the best forms of exercise there is.

The other good news is that there's a host of advantages to walking for people who have had back problems or want to avoid them. Obviously there's some impact on your spine involved, so you should talk to your practitioner before starting a walking program if you haven't done it before, but with most bad backs, walking can make things better.

Unlike a lot of other sports like cycling and many ball sports, your spine is upright the whole time you're walking. Your head, neck, shoulders, back, and hips should all be in vertical alignment as you cruise along. You use your legs to power you forward as you keep your upper body in balance, increasing blood flow (therefore oxygen!) to your muscles, tissues, and tendons, including those in your back.

Walking isn't the only exercise you should do if you want to keep your back in shape, but it's a good one to do in combination with some stretching and basic strengthening exercises. It's good for you in general because it's a great, safe, aerobic workout (which means it can help you lose weight if you want to) and of course it's easy, it's free, and it will keep you loose-limbed if you're doing it right.

If you've never done an aerobic workout before, start slowly, and work your way up in amount of time spent, and the speed you travel.

If you want to include walking as part of a routine to keep your back in shape, here's how you should do it:

Although you don't need to stretch all your muscle groups before you hit the road, it's not a bad idea to decompress your spine by hanging from a door or any stationary horizontal structure that will take all your weight. Even though it's gentle, walking has some impact on the spine, and you don't want to start out more squashed than you need to be.

Wear good shoes. Running shoes are the best, because they give you the support and cushioning you need. Once you've been walking a while, replace your shoes regularly. If your shoes lose their bounce, your spine will be the thing that absorbs the impact.

We hate the term "power walking." It's like "power dressing"—something for people more ambitious than we are. We like "fast walking" or "vigorous walking." Whatever you call it, to get a nice aerobic workout, you should walk faster than normal, but not so fast that you get dizzy or nauseous. It's good if you can walk fast enough to work up a sweat, but you're not out of breath once you stop.

The walking itself is easy. Don't worry about the length of your stride. It should be whatever is comfortable. As you walk, your foot should connect with the ground at the heel, then roll forward and push off at the toes. Don't land flat-footed or on the balls of your feet. Naturally, feet tend to turn out a little as we walk, but try to keep them somewhat parallel and hip width apart.

Let your upper body stay relaxed, with your shoulders loose and unhunched, and your arms swinging back and forth in the opposite direction of your legs on that side —which is the direction they usually go, in case you hadn't noticed. The great thing about the swinging motion is that the weight of your arms gently stretches your back and shoulder muscles, bringing them lots of oxygen. This motion can undo little knots you may have, and you'll be amazed how much better you'll feel.

Don't chop the air with your fists or keep your arms raised too high as you walk, because you'll miss out on that stretch. And don't carry hand-weights! This has become very popular lately, and is an example of multitasking at its dumbest. Weights can add to the impact and compression of your spine, which is what you want to minimize when you're walking. Do your weights at home or in the gym with your back in a protected position, preferably while you lie flat on the floor or against a backrest designed to take the load.

And don't carry a bottle of water (unless it's on a purpose-designed belt, with the bottle positioned in the center of your back). Carrying a water bottle is even worse than hand-weights, because it's just on one side, causing both compression and imbalance. Drink some water before you take your walk, and drink some more when you get back. It's not like you're running a marathon or heading off into the Mojave Desert for a week. We're talking about half an hour or so around the neighborhood. If you can't manage that without water, you need to see your doctor.

Even carrying a set of keys will tend to gradually imbalance you over some distance, so if you need to bring keys along, or you're carrying a Walkman, periodically change hands.

Let your hips roll when you walk. The catwalk thing may appear to be no more than a sexy come-on tactic, but it's actually a great way to exercise the muscles, ligaments, and joints in your lumbar and pelvic areas. Anyway, there's nothing wrong with sexy.

Some people like to wear those little monitors that display their pulse rate, as they help maintain their interest in what they're doing and are especially useful for cardiac patients. But if you're happy to work out without one, that's fine, as long as you use common sense. If you walk vigorously for around half an hour at least three times a week, your heart and lungs will thank you.

When it's possible, walk on soft surfaces like grass, dirt, or sand rather than tarmac or concrete, as long as your ankles and ligaments are strong enough. Remember, you want to minimize the impact of each step on your spine.

And keep to flat surfaces, or ones where there's a gentle incline. Avoid steep downhill paths.

Women should wear bras with sufficient support, both to prevent unnecessary strain on their upper backs, and to prevent microtearing and stretching of the breast tissue. Fast-walking braless is a bad look, but it will be even worse if you've been doing it for ten years.

Aerobic exercise is essential for all of us, and walking is a particularly good form of it for people with a history of back trouble. It's ideal for people with desk jobs because it increases blood flow to parts of your body that have been stagnating. It's stable, symmetrical, and relatively risk-free. Remember that you're not just getting an aerobic workout: you're conditioning your back-support muscles. So throw on your running shoes and go!

RUNNING

RUNNING ISN'T NECESSARILY bad for your back, but if you've had back trouble and want to run, you have to be careful. You need to have really well-developed abdominal muscles to support your back and minimize the impact as you go. Of course you shouldn't run with pain. But unless you have some major derangement of the spine like a herniated disc or degenerative osteoarthritis, running can actually be good for your back.

As with all other forms of exercise, talk to your practitioner about it. Because there is slightly more risk than with walking, you should probably get some coaching before you take off. The same general rules apply to running as to walking, about staying on grass or sand rather than concrete, and keeping your upper body relaxed as you go, but you really need someone to help you develop a technique so that you're not in danger of reinjury. Be even more cautious about running on uneven ground.

If you do get into running, and this applies to walking as

well, try to catch your reflection in shop or car windows as you go by. It's good to have an idea of your style and posture. You might be surprised at what you see. It's also smart to demonstrate your technique to your trainer or practitioner so they can recommend corrections that might help you keep your back in better shape.

SWIMMING AND AQUAEROBICS

Swimming is certainly the safest aerobic exercise, even more so than walking, because you're buoyed by the water and there's hardly any impact or compression on your spine; exercising in water is one of the best ways to strengthen and tone your back. After a severe injury, patients' first rehabilitation workout is often hydrotherapy. But a water workout can be as gentle or as vigorous as you like it.

All the traditional swimming strokes including freestyle, backstroke, breast stroke, and butterfly are fantastic exercises for your whole back and all the muscles we use to support the back. However, breaststroke and butterfly are not recommended if your back problem is aggravated by extension (back-bending movements). Backstroke is more benign, unless you also have shoulder strain. In any case, you can get a lot of benefits out of doing something as simple as walking through the water.

With the water at about waist-height, walk as briskly as you can through it, staying upright and not leaning forward. You'll find the resistance the water offers makes it a surprisingly challenging workout. The deeper the water, the harder it will get.

To exercise your abdominal, back, gluteal, and leg muscles, hold a small kickboard extended out in front of you, and floating on your tummy, kick your way up and down the lanes at the pool.

For more elaborate exercises you can enroll in various

classes that are held at most community pools. These days there's a wonderful range of courses, from basic swimming to advanced aquaerobics, and they're offered to everyone from infants to the elderly.

You might want to combine a water program with another form of exercise like walking or yoga as well as your basic back exercises. Even though it should be informed by your practitioner's advice, the program you go with is up to you.

WEIGHT TRAINING

DON'T BE SCARED off by the mistaken idea that weights will compress your spine. If done carefully and under supervision, weight training can strengthen your back muscles without having a negative impact. It can also build bone density and help fight osteoporosis.

It is absolutely essential that you talk to your practitioner before getting into weights. Even then, you should make an appointment with a trainer at your gym so he or she can show you what exercises are safe and how to do them. Then once you're doing them, you should still be periodically supervised.

Before you start, make sure you've been working on your abdominals. You don't want to start bench-pressing or doing shoulder lifts with weak tummy muscles, because you'll need them for support. Strong abs can prevent further back injury and help control your lifts.

The great thing about weight training is that you can target very specific areas that you want to work on. For example, you may have a particular weakness in your upper back that's causing those muscles to go into spasm just from minimal strain like hauling in the groceries or using a keyboard. You can tell your trainer this and be given a precise program to strengthen those muscles.

The trick is to start very slowly. At first you might think

that you aren't using enough weight to make a difference. But it's not just the weight; it's what the muscle is doing with the weight that builds strength in the right place. That, and the number of repetitions. What may feel like a really light weight at first will start feeling quite heavy after doing a movement twenty-five times. Remember to get your technique right first and increase resistance later.

The idea with weights is always to keep them stable. You get no benefit out of jerking an enormous weight that you're huffing and puffing and wobbling around with. Leave that to the guys who go for the medals. That's how your back could get into trouble, and is another reason to be supervised.

OTHER SPORTS

SAILING CAN BE surprisingly beneficial because the unpredictable movements of the boat or yacht cause you to make minor corrections in your back and abdominal muscles, thereby re-setting patterns of tension and restriction.

Cycling can be great because it strengthens lower back and abdominal muscles and it's also symmetrical, but it can be problematic depending on your history. With some back conditions, the bending forward is actually good because it opens up the vertebrae at the back where there might be the worst compression. In other cases, the forward bending might exacerbate a problem. There's also the issue of static loading on the upper back from having to hold your head and neck up as you lean forward. As with everything else, ask your practitioner about it first.

Racquet sports such as tennis and squash are great workouts but you have to be careful of the lopsided emphasis on your right or left, as well as the impact of sudden lateral movements. And of course the occasional running into a wall or a fence, or your opponent. If you've had a severe back injury, it's probably best for you to stick to things like swimming, yoga, weights, or walking.

Golf can be good for people with a history of back trouble, but only after recovery and when you've strengthened your abdominal muscles to help support your back while you swing.

A lot of people assume that horseback riding is probably not the wisest choice if you have back trouble because of the impact, but this isn't necessarily the case. Riders are trained to develop their back and abdominal muscles and maintain good lordosis to stabilize their movements and control the horse. So riding can actually be great for healthy backs, as long as you have proper training. Injuries occur more often when the rider doesn't have that upright control and bounces too forcefully in the saddle, leading to excessive compression. Just watch out for some of the other, more unpredictable variables. Like the horse.

Surfing, skiing, and snowboarding can be fabulous sports for people with healthy backs, because you use back and abdominal muscles to maintain balance. But because of their ballistic nature (you're moving under the force of gravity), there can also be significant risks.

Rowing and kayaking are very tricky workouts, and injuries to discs are common. The leaning forward motion (bending at the waist), with rowing in particular, can cause a round-shouldered, forward-leaning carriage and herniated discs, especially in the lumbar spine. Rowing machines that make you sit up straight, not lunging forward, and keep your movements symmetrical are actually great for your back, shoulder, and abdominal muscles. Watch out with forward-bending, side-pulling rowing. Surf lifesaving rowing crews commonly experience lower back problems because of this, and problems are emerging even among school rowing teams.

At the risk of stating the obvious, avoid contact sports.

With everything else, from rock-climbing to hang-gliding to bungee jumping, consult your practitioner and use common sense.

POST-WORKOUT STRETCH

WE KNOW WE'VE said this before, but remember to stretch after every kind of workout. (We're trying to brainwash you, so bear with us.) You may feel loose and like you don't need a stretch, but once you've stopped your activity and your body has started cooling down, the muscles you've been using will start to contract unless you extend them. This is also why it's so important to throw on a sweater or warm-up jacket after you exercise. Do that as soon as you finish your activity and keep it on while you're stretching.

If you've had back trouble in the past, make sure you do some back stretches even if you don't think you've really used those muscle groups. You use your back for everything even if it doesn't seem like it.

MAGNESIUM AND CALCIUM

A WELL-BALANCED diet that includes lots of fruits and vegetables will give us most of the vitamins, minerals, and other nutrients we need to maintain good health. But we don't always have a well-balanced diet, and certain supplements are especially important when it comes to good backs.

Magnesium is indispensable in the maintenance of healthy muscles. Anyone who works out needs a lot of it, so you may need a supplement in the form of tablets or a powder you can mix in drinks or food. As we get older we need more—especially women.

Make sure you talk to your practitioner or the naturopath at your health food shop to find out if you should be taking more than the minimum recommended on the packaging, which is often the case if you get frequent muscle spasms or you suffer from a condition such as fibromyalgia.

The same goes for calcium. We need more as we age because we lose bone density, and usually we don't get enough in our diets to compensate for the natural losses.

CROUCHING TIGERS, BENDING DRAGONS:
Ergonomics and Your Environment

*O*kay, **so now** you've fixed your bad back, you're a yoga maniac, and everything will be peachy, right? Well, it can be, but there's one challenge left. The small matter of working and living. You need to make sure of two things. One—that your work, home, and play environments aren't conspiring to bring pain back; and two—that the way you move within those environments is the right way to move.

The word "ergonomics" comes from two Greek words: ergo, which means work, and nomoi, which means natural laws. So ergonomics is the study of how natural laws—like bio-mechanics and physics—relate to how we work. When we say "work" we don't just mean how we earn a living. We mean doing anything, from opening a window to picking up a baby, where we use our bodies in relation to the world around us.

How our bodies do what they do is often the reason that our backs went haywire in the first place. So in this section, we're going to give you lots of great, realistic ideas on how to improve your everyday movement habits to prevent re-injury.

LIFTING

REMEMBER WE MENTIONED that our backs are only designed to last around thirty years—the approximate life span of our cave-dwelling ancestors? Well not only that, but it's been estimated that modern man does ten times more lifting than our neo-lithic counterparts. And a lot of the time, we lift badly.

One of the most common ways that people injure their backs is lifting. You might be a builder with a load of bricks or a child with a backpack, but whatever it is you're lifting, the outcome is often the same: back pain, usually in that vulnerable lumbar area.

The professional costs are astronomical. The most common reason for being absent from work is injury due to lifting and carrying. Builders, movers, and nurses are among the most common victims, and sometimes there's no way around it. But often there is.

There is a right way to lift so that you can protect your back and get the job done. Just follow these rules.

- ◆ Plan your lift beforehand and visualize your movements.
- ◆ Never bend from the waist, unless you have to. Instead, crouch or squat as low as you can, bending your knees and hips, keeping your back as upright as possible.
- ◆ If possible, start with the load between your feet, which should be hip-width apart.
- ◆ Hold the load close to your body—ideally right up against it.
- ◆ Breathe in deeply and engage your abdominal muscles as you move. (It's that internal airbag effect that weight-lifters use.)

- When you're breathing out, do it slowly to protect your discs.
- Tilt up slowly to get a good grip, but don't rock backward.
- Keep your elbows tucked into your sides.
- Rise using your leg and gluteal muscles.
- Don't twist your spine as you go.
- Wear low-heeled shoes or boots with nonslip soles and ankle support.
- Wear gloves if they'll make it easier to grip your load.
- Don't carry a load in one hand if you can carry it in two.
- If the load is really heavy, get someone to lift it with you and make sure your movements are in sync.
- If you can't lift the load safely on your own or even with help, get other people to do it or call for the forklift. There's a time to be macho and a time to be smart. This is the latter.

These rules don't just apply to lifting heavy loads. We're talking about lifting a shoe off the floor. Or a dropped coin. Any time at all that you need to lower yourself to do or get something, take a second to think about what you're doing, then crouch or squat rather than bend from the waist. Keep your spine vertical as much as possible. Think crouching tiger, not bending dragon.

BEDS

WE MENTIONED THIS spot (where you spend a third of your life!) in the Do-it-Yourself chapter, but that was just in relation to dealing with current pain. Even if you don't have back pain now, you can help prevent it by sleeping on a firm mattress. Not only will you sleep better, you'll wake up happier, sex will be better (seriously!), and you can kiss soreness and muscle spasms good-bye.

Firm, high-quality mattresses don't come cheap, but think of all the money you'll save by not going to the doctor, buying drugs, or missing out on work! And make sure it's big enough, especially if you share your bed. You're more likely to sleep in awkward positions and cramp up if you're being elbowed to the edge by one of those people who jumps hurdles while asleep. And you know how, when you buy a new mattress, the label says to turn it around and flip it over every once in a while, and you never have? Well, start. The internal structures of a mattress are vulnerable to compression in the same way your back is, and you can even out the stresses if you change the spots you stick into.

Futons are nice and firm, but they can get too hard (and yes, there is such a thing as too hard) if you don't follow the instructions about rolling them and flipping them periodically. This can be a little tough to do, especially if you have a tricky back and you have to toss around a double, queen, or king.

So think carefully about what kind of mattress will suit you and then open your wallet wide.

In an earlier section we talked about good ways to lie in bed, and they still apply, even once your pain has gone. Use a cushion between your knees (while lying on your side) for lower back stability, and only one smallish or medium-size pillow under your head to prevent neck and shoulder strain that can eventually have a ripple effect and work its way down your spine. Some people find that those orthopedic pillows with raised edges for neck support help them, but others can experience dreadful pain, so borrow one and try it before you shell out.

On your back, slide a pillow or two under your knees if you really want to feel like royalty. Some people are in love with those long body pillows that you have kind of snaking under and in front of you, and while they look cool, they can tend to get in the way and not travel with you when you roll over. But if it works for you, go for it.

If you find that you tend to roll on to your tummy in your sleep, stop that by placing a pillow against your chest and stomach when you're on your side.

In the Do-it-Yourself chapter we explained how to get out of bed, and this applies whether you're in pain or not. Think prevention! Roll onto your side facing the edge of the bed and use your arms and hands to push yourself up as you gently swing your legs to the floor. As you do this, engage your tummy muscles, and then rise with both feet evenly planted on the floor at the same time. Reverse the sequence to get in.

With babies' cribs, you definitely want to keep the mattresses low enough so they can't climb out, but with newborns this is less of an issue. So while you can still get away with it, keep your infant's mattress on the highest rung so you don't have to bend too far at the waist to pick the little one up.

LIVING ROOM FURNITURE

THIS ONE'S EASY. Don't have couches and chairs (more about those scoundrels later) that give way under your buttocks or cave in when you lean back. The seat cushions and backrests of living room furniture should be as firm as your mattress. Especially if you spend more than twenty minutes at a time in front of that talking box in the corner.

If you do have some cave-in-at-the-back furniture, use throw cushions to support your back. Or, you may have a couch or chair whose seat is deeper than the length of your thighs, so you have to slouch to lean against the backrest. This is where those throw cushions will come in handy again. Your lower back should always be well supported so you get a nice little inward curve.

Remember that the point of living rooms is to lounge, not to get your back and neck in terrible knots.

STAIRS

WHEN YOU WALK up stairs, plant your whole foot on the step, not just the front half. Going up on your toes and balls of your feet is hard on your knees and can induce pelvic instability. It's easier to keep balanced on your whole foot.

If you have back trouble, that banister is a real help. Hold on as you go up or down, and take some of the pressure off your back as you make relatively unstable (and impossible to avoid) movements. If there's an elevator, take it until you've recovered.

HOUSEWORK, GARDENING, AND A LITTLE GROOMING

IT SHOULDN'T HAVE to be said, but from personal experience, we know it does: when you have a bad back, don't do housework! You may think civilization will fall if you don't change the sheets or scrub the shower floor, but it won't. Always give yourself enough recovery time before you tackle the cleaning, and even then, use preventative measures to keep your back happy.

Bed-making

One of the things you have to get over when you commit to getting rid of bad habits is being embarrassed about looking silly. Just keep reminding yourself that you'd look even sillier in traction. Or hunched over a walker at the age of forty-two.

A lot of housework involves bending over or leaning forward at the waist, and as we know by now, that's the worst thing you can do for your lower back, especially when you do it over and over again. So when you make the beds or change the sheets, see how much of it you can do on your knees. We know, it conjures up images of indentured servitude, but once you try it you'll realize how much less bending is involved, and how much less exhausting that is. Especially the tucking-in part, when you half lift the mattress. This is so much easier to do from a kneeling or crouching position. If your floors are carpeted you're lucky, and if not, wear pants.

Other cleaning

The rule of thumb is simply, unless you have to, don't bend from the waist. Instead, crouching, kneeling, or squatting might be just the thing if you have to dust the skirting boards, clean the bath, scrub bathroom tiles, clean low cupboards, etc.

Sinks and countertops

Most sinks and countertops are installed too low for the average-size adult. And tall people are really at a disadvantage! Well, we have seen some modern kitchens where somebody has the right idea, but they're rare. In most homes, the kitchen and bathroom sinks and counters are set at a level where kids can use them, which is great if you're nine. But it means that the rest of us have to bend at the waist for jobs like preparing food, doing the dishes, handwashing clothes, washing faces, washing hands, and of course . . . cleaning the sinks and countertops!

The problem is that most of us are not in a position to run out and order a quick bathroom and kitchen renovation, and of course some of us have kids, and we don't want them to have to wash their hands in the toilet. Fortunately, there is a solution.

Ideally, a sink should be at the same height as your waist. So you have to be inventive and compensate for the difference between the ideal and the real. If you have the space, keep a tub or large bowl next to the sink to do the dishes and hand-washing in. Or if you are using a low sink, pick up the item to be washed and straighten your back while you wash it. It's better to lift something up to waist-height (especially when it's light like a glass or plate) than to bend down to it. So many of the bad habits we have we don't really need.

When you brush your teeth and you have to lean over the sink, support yourself with one hand resting on the sink edge to remove the load from your lower back.

Don't wash or dye your hair in the sink. Not unless some-one is holding a gun to your head. You have to bend so far forward at the waist for this task that the load you put on your lumbar spine should be illegal. Even if it seems like more trouble at the time, the shower is the only place for this kind of hair maintenance.

With a low kitchen countertop, put a thick butcher block or cutting board on top of it to get your work surface closer to waist-height for food preparation. Or—and this is lateral thinking at its simplest—sit on a low stool so that you lower the height of your waist to match the countertop. Or do as much as you can sitting at the kitchen or dining room table, if that height's better.

In a garage or a greenhouse, counters are also often too low. The trick here is to put a brick or two under each of the legs to raise the surface.

Windows and garage doors

If your back is acting up, be very careful raising or lower-ing windows and garage doors. They often get stuck and you really have to exert some force to move them. When you do that, most of the pressure is exerted on your spine. It's really just another form of lifting. So if you have pain caused by compression or associated trouble like a herniated disc, leave the window or door where it is or get someone else to do it.

But even when you're pain-free, make sure you get as close to the window or door as possible to move it up or down.

Don't wash the windows with a bad back. Raising your arms above the normal range could make matters worse, and the repetitive motion required when you're getting that extra shiny translucence is just the thing you don't need.

Gardening

It sounds so pleasant. So harmless. Gardening—spending time out among the flowers and trees, the birds and the bees, caring for your lovely growing things while you relax in the sunshine.

In fact, gardening is a minefield of potential back disasters. Accidents waiting to happen. Disc deathtraps. But you can avoid them all, if you're smart.

A lot of gardening seems to demand you bend at the waist. But you could do many of those jobs while you crouch, kneel, squat, or even sit cross-legged if you can manage that comfortably. Weeding, planting, fertilizing, and digging are all things you can do in these positions. You can also use long-handled tools so you can do some work in a standing position.

Be very careful when moving pots filled with soil. Instead of lifting and carrying a full pot, try tilting it to the side and rolling it on the ground slowly along its bottom rim. You should be able to manage this without tipping out the plant or its soil.

One of the most basic ways to protect your back while you garden, or in fact anything that involves repetitive movement, is to rest often, and change your activity (or rather the position of your activity) frequently. It's that identical twisting or bending motion over a period of time that tends to shear away at discs and other structures. So intersperse some low-level weeding with some standing-level pruning when you can. If you currently have a bad back or are recovering from one, it's probably best to avoid gardening altogether. Especially digging, which has to involve some bending as well as lifting.

Renovations

If you're going to be brave and do your own home improvements, congratulations. You'll save money and feel more proud of the results. Just don't pay with the health of your back. Like gardening, renovation work such as painting, sanding, and tiling involves a lot of repetitive work that you have to get your back into.

So remember to bend from the waist as little as you can, and squat, sit, or stand instead. Stop and rest often—every ten minutes or so—even just to stand back and admire your handiwork. Change your position as frequently as possible. And change your activity every once in a while too. The muscles, ligaments, and joints you use to paint the ceiling are not all the same ones you use to lay floor tiles. So shuffle your work schedule and save your back.

Grocery shopping

A common back injury occurs when someone decides to challenge the Olympic weight-lifting record and carry eight full bags of groceries from the shop or the car all the way home. This is dumb for so many reasons, but we've all done it. (Well, we have anyway.)

All it takes to avoid this problem is a little planning and a little patience. If you're walking any distance, you should only carry a couple of bags at a time. What this means is that if you're on foot, you need to shop either every day or every couple of days. On your way home from work, pick up what you need for dinner and the next day. Then if you have room in your allotted two bags to carry some more, think ahead and get things you'll soon need to save yourself a trip next time.

If you do one of those big weekly shopping trips by car, and have more than you can comfortably carry home in one go, just bring in a few bags at first with the things that need to go in the fridge. They usually bag them separately anyway. Sometimes you can get away with just one trip the first time around if you only take in the things you need right away or that would spoil if left behind. You can leave canned goods, paper products, and other things in the trunk, and get them later when you have to use the car again. Or, if you want to unpack everything right away, just accept the fact that making one or two or even three trips is smarter and less painful than trying to do it all at once. Look at it as your aerobic workout for the day. And carry the bags with the handles hanging as close as possible to the palms of your hands, not your fingertips. You can take more weight that way, and your load is more stable.

FASHION ACCESSORIES

Shoes

Probably the most awful truth regarding back care is that high heels aren't good for you. We agree: it's not fair. They look so absolutely fabulous. But what they do—and this is more true the higher they are—is force your hips to tip forward creating an unnatural and extreme arch in your lumbar spine. This can lead to all sorts of problems from disc trouble to misalignment of internal organs. Not to mention sore feet!

But we're not going to tell you to throw away those brand new red stilettos. We're not that mean. The idea is that, as with a lot of other vices, high heels can be all right in moderation. So minimize the damage by following a few guidelines.

Don't wear high heels if you're in the throes of a back attack. You'll merely be prolonging your agony. Be daring and wear flat sandals with that evening gown.

Wear your high heels for a few hours, but not all day and night. The longer you inflict that strange posture on your spine, the likelier an injury is.

If you wear your heels to a party, kick them off when you have a dance. People will think you're just a free-spirited party animal and not a responsible carer for the health of your back.

Standing around in your high heels is one thing, but try not to walk for any distance in them. From the limo to the red carpet is fine, but across town is not. Each time you take a step, your weight shifts from one side to the other, potentially throwing out of balance the structures of your back. If this imbalance is inflicted while your hips are tipped forward and your lumbar spine awkwardly arched, the risk of injury is greater.

When you take your high heels off after wearing them for a while, lie on the floor and do a nice knees-to-chest stretch where you curve your spine in the opposite direction it's just been forced into. It will feel great and can reverse some of the effects of the previous few hours' torture.

The sad fact is that flat shoes are good for you. But if you work on your feet you probably already know that. You don't see waitresses or nurses or factory workers in stilettos. And not only are flats better for you, so are soft soles.

Unglamorous they may be, but sneakers or any flat shoes with rubber soles can help prolong the life and health of your back. Think about it. Every time you take a step you send a shock wave up through your spine. Every step has a compressive impact. Be nice to yourself and cushion that impact with the right shoes. Or, when you have to wear your three-inch heels just for a few hours, slip in some of those soft insoles you can buy at the pharmacy. They'll make a difference not by correcting your posture but by softening the blows to your skeleton. Every little bit helps.

Hand and shoulder bags

It should be pretty obvious by now that balance is one of the keys to a happy back. So it should be equally obvious that a heavy bag carried on one side can pull your spine and nearby muscles and ligaments off center. So when you carry a bag, whether on your shoulder or in your hand, change sides frequently to keep evening the tension.

Unless somebody's life depends on it (somebody you like a lot), don't weight your bag down with lots of unnecessary items. This is common with moms who bring half the nursery with them when they go out. Next time, make sure you bring only the essentials.

The sorry fact is that even nonmoms tend to bring too much with them when they leave the house. Perfume bottle, a makeup case containing forty-seven components only three of which they use through the day, cell phone, wallet, address book or palm pilot, pens, check book, keys, hairbrush, tampons, pads, condoms, books, and a host of other arcane artifacts all find their way regularly into a woman's bag. And often the bag itself is the size of a small steamer trunk and made of leather, so it's heavy. Next time you go out, go through your bag and fish out anything you won't need. We bet a lot of you can halve the weight of your bag without missing a thing.

Also consider using a bag in a lighter-weight fabric like microfiber.

With a shoulder bag, it's great if you can carry it across your body, with the strap on one shoulder and the bag itself resting against the opposite side. This means putting the strap over your head, but it's not that bad a look, and you'll be amazed at how much easier it is to tote around.

If you have just a small amount to carry, use your pockets or one of those fanny bags. Okay, so they're not the most glamorous fashion accessory, but they're practical.

BABY TRANSPORT

WHEN IT COMES to your baby, try to apply the rules for lifting and carrying already mentioned. A common injury can occur when a mother carries her baby on one hip, forcing her spine into an awkward curve, and putting uneven weight on the back and pelvis. So if you can, keep the weight of the baby as centered as possible.

When it comes to carriers, it's a personal thing, but you have to think of your back and not just your baby. Front-packs are nice because they keep you and your baby close to each other, but they can be hard to put on without putting undue strain on your back. Once you've got them on, they're fine with newborns, but as your baby puts on weight—which infants do so quickly!—it can lead to serious strain on your back, neck, and shoulders.

Back carriers, where the baby sits in a canvas seat attached to a lightweight frame you wear strapped on like a backpack, give the baby a wonderful view of the world but can be hard on your poor back. The weight of the baby is farther away from your body than with a front-pack, and there's also more room for him or her to squirm suddenly, shifting its weight and throwing your back into unexpected places. These carriers should only be worn if you're strong, have taut abs, and the baby doesn't weigh too much, as spinal compression is inevitable. And never wear them for long periods.

Slings, which women have been using for centuries, are actually very efficient, and you can periodically shift the position of the baby to spread the weight and minimize strain.

With regard to your back, the safest mode of baby transport is certainly the stroller. Not only do you not bear the weight of your child, you can hang light bags of groceries from the handles or in the basket.

Once your pride and joy learns to walk, resist his or her constant, helpless cries to be picked up and carried. Hard though it may be, your resolve here will stand you in good stead throughout your parenting years.

PHONES

DON'T TALK ON the phone with the handset cradled between your ear and your shoulder if you don't have a free hand. Not even for a few minutes. That can be enough to send tense neck and shoulder muscles into spasm, and of course there's that old domino effect that can be deadly in the case of phone cramp.

If you have to talk on the phone while using your hands for something else (like driving, cooking, changing diapers, changing tires, typing, applying nail polish, or any of the other hundred things we do when we multitask), use a hands-free speaker or head set. Or—and this is novel thought—hang up and call back later.

DRIVING

CAR SEATS ARE designed better than they used to be, but you often still don't get enough lumbar support. You can compensate by having a little cushion or a folded towel or jacket that you put right behind your waist. They even make supports specially designed for this purpose. They're great to use on trips of any length, and can help prevent bad backs, neck strain, and headaches.

Keep your seat far enough forward so that you can move your foot from the brake to the accelerator and back without lifting your whole leg. Same with the foot you use for the clutch if you drive a manual. Try it now and feel how much strain there is on your lower back when you lift one leg even a few centimeters off the ground. Most people have their driver's seats way too far back, and are not even aware of the unnecessary stress they're putting on their backs. You should be able to depress each of the pedals and still have your knees bent. When you can do this, adjust your seat so that you can also hold the top of the steering wheel and still have a slight bend at your elbows.

Before you go on a long trip, and when you stop periodically in the middle of one, do a few stretches to loosen things up. Some gentle twists or rotations of the neck and back will counteract the effects of your rigid, front-facing posture as well as the muscle tension that comes from the mental stress of driving, especially at high speeds. If you tend to get sciatica, you'll be a much happier camper if you do some gluteal and hamstring stretches before you take the wheel. Then do the same exercises again once you get there.

Especially if you have a bad back, turning the wheel without power steering can be torture, so go for power steering with your next car purchase, or investigate a trade-in. If this is a bit of an extravagant solution, at least pump your front tires to the highest limit given by the manufacturer and check the pressure regularly. You'll be amazed how much easier it is to steer.

When you get in and out of the car, don't do it one foot at a time. You may think the right way looks or feels weird at first, but after a while you'll swear by it. It's the same principle as getting in and out of bed. To get in, back in with your buttocks first, sit down with both your feet planted next to the car, then swing them inside together. For getting out, reverse it: swing your legs around and plant them on the ground, then get up like you're getting out of a chair, and use the door for support if you want to. If it makes it easier for your knees to clear the steering wheel, move the seat back before you get out. Always maintain a balance between the right and left sides of your body when you can. Think of what an unbalanced movement you make when you do the whole thing on one leg. And guess what—it's completely unnecessary.

FLYING

AS EVERYBODY KNOWS, sitting in a cramped space, such as an economy class seat on an airplane, isn't all that comfortable. But when the flight is a long one, like from the U.S. to Australia, Asia, or Europe, your back can really feel the pinch.

When you buy your ticket for one of those marathon trips, book an aisle seat at the same time. This way, you can get up and walk around the cabin without having to climb over your fellow passengers. Once you're up, do some stretches. If you don't feel comfortable about doing them in the aisle or at the back where your audience is smaller, you can always do a little workout in the toilets. Find the one that has the pull-down baby-changing table in it. It's bigger than the others and you'll have enough room to do some nice deep stretches before returning to your seat.

Stretching and movement will also have the added bonus of reducing fluid buildup around the ankles.

It's also a good idea to do some stretching at the gate before you get on the plane. We have a friend who does this before he heads overseas. While he always gets a few funny looks, he's the one laughing as he gets off the plane feeling nice and limber, and the rest of them are hunched over and grisly, looking like that bell ringer from Notre Dame.

A word about luggage. Most people pack too much when they travel, and end up wearing the same few things instead of the entire wardrobe they brought with them. And of course that wardrobe and the Cadillac-sized suitcase it comes in weigh a ton. Even if you have porters to help you, or you use a luggage cart, there are always moments when you've got to do the lugging yourself. So next trip, pack light and do your back a favor. And big or small, always buy luggage with wheels. The ones with the retractable handles are particularly good because they minimize the amount of bending you have to do.

THE OFFICE

BELIEVE IT OR not, this is an even more dangerous environment than the garden. It may not look threatening, but it's full of traps that people fall into because they don't know how to use their bodies in relation to their furniture and equipment. And sometimes the furniture and equipment are to blame.

Computers

Computers have revolutionized our lives. Because they make the exchange of information quicker and easier, they've brought people closer together. But not physically. The impact of computers and IT (information technology) on people's physical health is just beginning to be understood. And the news is scary.

When it comes to our bodies, IT might also be called Inertia Training. Working in an office was never something that promoted great physical conditioning, but at least in the old days, people would get up from their desks and go to another office down the hall or on another floor to talk to one another.

Or they might walk to the copy machine and even run into someone there.

But nowadays, technology does more while you do less. Instead of making copies of documents like memos to distribute around the office, you email your coworkers. Instead of going to the mailroom to send external documents, you e-mail. Instead of walking down the hall to chat to the boss or your secretary, you e-mail.

The inertia associated with being attached to our computers

is causing us to lose strength and mobility in our backs. And the effects are cumulative and can be long term.

In recent surveys, between two-thirds and three-quarters of all office workers report pain or discomfort, and they blame their computers. Hand and arm ailments, as well as neck and back strain and stiffness account for most of it. This used to be called RSI (repetitive strain injury), but is now referred to as OOS (occupational overuse syndrome.) Experts predict that OOS will become epidemic in the next decade. From where we're sitting, it already is. Symptoms can range from mild discomfort to constant, debilitating pain that could ultimately prevent you from working for a substantial amount of time.

But don't despair! There are measures you can take to keep from becoming a victim, or to turn things around if you already are.

We'll get to the wicked laptop in a minute but first we'll look at the good old desktop computer. Many people have it in the wrong position. Here are the rules:

- The computer should be directly in front of you, not to the side.
- The top of the screen should be at eye level.
- The keyboard should sit at elbow height, and if possible, be angled slightly toward you.
- There should be sufficient surface between you and the keyboard to rest your wrists on while you're typing.
- You shouldn't rely too much on your mouse, and instead use your keyboard as much as you can.
- Position your mouse as close to your body as you can.
- Your feet should be flat on the floor and your legs bent at a 90-degree angle.

The reasons for these rules all relate to back care, not to mention the health of your hands, wrists, and elbows. If your computer is off to one side, you do lots of repetitive twisting, which your muscles and discs won't like. If your screen is too low, you need to tilt your head down to read it, and this creates a static load, or unmoving weight on your upper spine. If your keyboard lies flat rather than being angled, this loading is increased because you have to tilt your head and lean forward. The weight of your head is easiest to balance if it rests on your spine with you looking straight ahead. Your keyboard should be at elbow level so that your shoulders aren't hunched up as you type. The muscles, ligaments, and vertebrae of your upper back are more relaxed if your upper arms can hang vertically. You need to be able to rest your wrists while you type because otherwise you're holding the whole weight of your arms and hands in the air as you type. This is more static loading on your spine and nearby structures. It's exhausting and compressive. And finally, overuse of the mouse destabilizes your back because it's static loading on one side, as you extend your arm and perform fine movements with your hand, creating a curve or twist in your spine and overuse of the muscles on that side.

There are desks specially designed to set your computer components at the right levels, but most people don't use them and sometimes they're impractical. What this means is that often monitors just sit on the desk behind the keyboard, which is way too low. All you need to do to correct this is to get a box or a stand of some kind—even a phonebook will do—to sit your monitor on. You can then adjust your chair height so that the desk itself is even with your elbows. This probably means that you're sitting pretty high and can't cross your legs, but that's better for you anyway!

When you have notes to copy or work from, clip them to a vertical stand so that they're around the same height as your monitor. And move them from one side of the monitor to the other every ten minutes or so to keep your neck from repeating a twist in one direction.

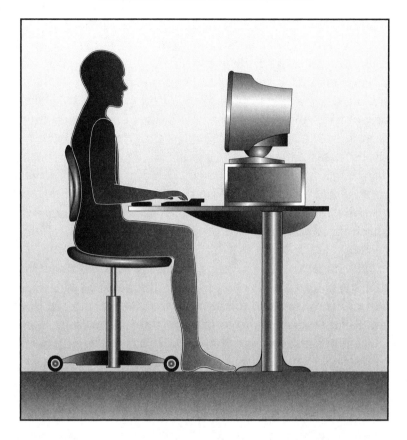

When computers went portable they made life easier in one way, but harder on our backs. For a start, even the slimmest "notebooks" or "laptops" are still pretty heavy, especially when you're lugging them around with their connecting wires in their own carry bag. They're usually dangling from one shoulder while in transit, which is the worst way they could be carried. But their "portability" isn't their biggest problem. The really nasty stuff happens once you've opened them up on the desk or table in front of you. Or even worse, on your lap!

There's no way you can arrange a laptop so that you can have good posture. If the screen is high enough (eye-level), then your hands are up around your chin. If the keyboard is low enough (elbow-height), then your head has to hang at a neck-tearing forty-five degree angle. Either way, you've got a huge amount of static load on your spine, and your muscles are being asked to perform completely unnecessary and tiring tasks. And because you can't angle the keyboard, it's hard to rest your wrists while you type, and you have to lean over further to see it.

You can, of course, adapt your laptop so that at the office you use it with a separate keyboard and mouse, and this is a good solution if you don't want to be constantly copying files from one computer to another, or if you can only afford one computer.

The problem is that laptops were originally designed for short-term use—on planes, in hotel rooms, on trains on the way to meetings—and for short-term use, they're great. But what a lot of people do is use their laptops full-time, instead of alternating them with their desktops, because it's more convenient to have all their files in one computer. Now we have handheld computers—teeny little state-of-the-art machines the size and thickness of a cigarette case. Hopefully people won't replace their laptops with these little toys: but if they do, no doubt they'll call it progress.

Chairs and sitting

No matter how good our chairs are, we have to face the fact that sitting in chairs is unnatural. Squatting causes less stress on the spine and can be done for longer periods. Our ancestors squatted or sat cross-legged, and every society that still does so has many fewer cases of bad backs than the rest of us. Chairs are another example of how the so-called civilized alternative is actually not civilized at all.

But chairs are here to stay, and luckily there are ways to sit on them and protect your back. And of course some chairs are better for your back than others.

You want to sit up straight while maintaining that nice little inward curve at the base of your back instead of slouching with your back compressed and your shoulders curved forward. To help you do this, there are really good ergonomically designed chairs that have terrific lumbar support, but even then you might need a little extra something like a cushion or a folded towel. And if you're using just any old straight-backed or slouch-backed chair, load the cushions in the right places for comfort and support. Slumping is one of those things that feels right, but actually it's just habit. Habit dulls our senses; because we've been sitting a certain way for a long time, our brain doesn't even notice that it's not comfortable anymore. It may seem comfortable for a while, but eventually your neck, shoulders, and back pay the price, whereas keeping the right curves in your spine reduces pressure on the discs.

If you use a chair all day at work, it's really important to get a good one. One of the other nifty things a proper ergonomic chair can do is lean back a little. Sometimes this feels great, especially with a little footrest to slightly elevate your feet. It's always good to redistribute your weight, even for just a short time.

Your chair should definitely have armrests! It's great to have somewhere to drape your arms or rest your elbows and forearms to take some of the load off your spine, and they're useful when changing positions or getting up to distribute more of the rising load. Ergonomic chairs also swivel, which is important so that you're not constantly twisting your spine to deal with paperwork or the phone on one side of your computer. Most of them come on casters too, which gives you another way of changing your position without taxing your back.

Those kneeling chairs can be good because they take most of your body weight through your knees rather than your lower spine like conventional chairs. These are the chairs that have the seat angled forward and then a platform for your knees angled back. They can take some getting used to, but they're good because they make it very hard to slouch. In most models, there's no backrest to lean on, so you have to sit up pretty straight and hold your tummy in to maintain the posture. But they have no armrests and can get a little tiring on your knees, so we like to alternate them with good ergonomic chairs with lumbar support and armrests.

Then there are those inflatable balls you can sit on. These have become very popular, and they certainly add some color to the office. They work on a similar principle to the kneeling chairs but are more versatile because you can use them to do various back exercises too. When using a ball as a chair, you have to keep your abdominal muscles as well as your leg muscles engaged to stay upright and maintain your balance. Some people find them too tiring as they give no back or arm support but others swear by them and use nothing else. Probably about half of your working day would be great, especially if you regularly take breaks and use them for some stretching.

Try not to cross your legs for too long while you're sitting as this unbalances your spine and pelvis. It also cuts off your circulation. And if do cross your legs, reverse their positions frequently.

There are several well-designed back supports that you can ask your practitioner or even a pharmacist about, and these devices can really help people who spend a lot of their days sitting at a desk. One of them is a simple system of straps that go around your waist like a belt and then hook around each knee, so that you sit up straight and have a nice little arch in your lumbar region. Just don't use them instead of exercising your back and abdominals. As a complement, they're fine.

Moving around

You can have the latest groovy ergonomic office equipment and still slump in your seat and compress your spine.

Your posture needs to be good and you should be in good enough shape to maintain the right posture, but even then sometimes it's hard because of our old friend, inertia.

Even perfect posture, if held for too long, will cause aches and pains. That's because we're meant to be moving around, not sitting inert, like robots. We're made of flesh and blood and we need to keep it all pumping! So the first thing you want to remember is to move around every once in a while. We know someone who uses the timer on her watch to beep every twenty minutes to remind her to roll her shoulders back a few times, arch her back, do some neck stretches. There's nothing better than staring at a computer monitor for ages to give you a really stiff neck.

Those exercises are fine for your upper body, but to decompress your spine try these:

Sitting in your chair, bend down with your head between your knees (holding on to your desk or the floor or other support as you lower yourself) and you'll get a great simple spinal stretch. Then, if your backrest is low enough, arch your back over the rear of your chair so you can lace the fingers of your hands together. At least a few times a day, especially if you've had back pain before, get on the floor and do some proper spinal stretches. And do a good, deep squat. And hang from a door. Or lie back on your inflated ball and get a nice stretch that way. Don't be embarrassed. Be the first. Start a trend.

And then boldly go where no man has gone before—or at least for a while—walk down the hall and talk to someone instead of e-mailing. Or just walk around the office pretending you're on a mission of some kind. You'll be more convincing if you have some papers in your hand. Most of you will always have something you can do away from your desk anyway. However you decide to do it, just get up and use your whole body for a few minutes at least every hour. The time you spend doing this you will gain back tenfold by not having to take days off work for having a bad back.

Some enlightened companies—and we're happy to say their number is growing—actually train their employees in good ergonomic practices and supply them with the right workstations to protect their health. This is smart thinking because it's the right thing to do and of course it also saves the company money in the long run. Less absenteeism and a happier, less exhausted workforce means greater productivity. Everybody wins.

De-stressing

One of the most important weapons against workplace back pain is the ability to unwind on the job, not just afterward. While you're sitting at your desk, your posture may be good but your muscles can be rigid and tense. Learn how to listen to your body and undo spots where tension has built up causing muscles to contract. A lot of us concentrate our tension in the shoulders and neck, and sometimes all it takes is to be aware of it and you can let go, allowing the head to move more freely. It helps to take a few deep breaths. You can even try closing your eyes for a few minutes.

Other people transfer their stress to their arms and hands, and it helps to consciously relax those parts of your body. Try to tap the keyboard and move the mouse lightly, rather than with tense, vigorous movements.

At lunchtime, sometimes it's easier to eat at your desk because you have so much to do, but that means that you haven't given yourself a chance to let go of tension that's accumulated through the morning. So even if you eat at your desk, take ten or twenty minutes to walk around the block or to wander around the shops or a park just to get your mind off work. Get some sun. Take in some air (even if it is a little polluted). You'll feel refreshed physically and mentally, and you'll be much better equipped to face the rest of the day.

Alexander Technique and Feldenkrais are great ways to figure out what you're doing wrong in your everyday life, especially at work, that may be causing back pain. Try to organize a visit from an Alexander or Feldenkrais teacher to your office for you and your colleagues. You can even get the boss to spring for the cost when you explain that good habits will increase productivity and decrease absenteeism!

KIDS

Computers

Back problems in children used to be a rarity. There were the few with scoliosis and other dysfunctions they were born with, but in general, because they hadn't joined the workforce, children's backs were unmarred by lifting injuries or OOS. All that has changed.

Things started going wrong when they changed the ergonomic design of school desks. In the old days, kids' desks were angled toward them, like draftsmen's tables. This meant that they could maintain a straight back while reading or writing, and their heads weren't tipped forward over their work. But now desks are flat, so they have to curve their spines and shoulders over their books, and dangle their heads above them to see what they're doing. This puts a terrific amount of static loading on their upper and middle spine, and encourages unnatural curvature. It also exerts more pressure on the lower back where cumulative damage can start nice and young while their bones are still forming.

And then we gave them computers. It's been great for our kids to be able to access so much information so easily. Most of them have been taught how to use basic programs in elementary school, and the Internet for researching their projects. But we don't know of many kids who were taught proper keyboard use, or how to set up their workstations for the best ergonomic outcome.

If you think grown-ups are lazy about posture, check out the way kids sit at a computer. Often, especially if they're playing a game, hours can go by with them in the same, forward slumping position. We may be breeding technological wizards, but they might also be the first entire generation of hunchbacks. Okay, that might be an over-statement, but the point is that our children are experiencing cumulative trauma to their musculoskeletal systems and in most cases they don't even feel it yet.

Some studies suggest that up to 30 percent of school kids are already showing signs of physical trauma attributable to computer use. And of course because they're glued to their keyboards it means they're not outside playing. The recent rise in obesity among children has also been blamed partly on computer use, which has compounded the problems already created by television.

The frightening thing is that we're only just beginning to see the effects of mass postural dysfunction among young people who grew up with computers, and no large-scale studies have yet been done. Some experts in the fields of ergonomics and other physical sciences recommend that children not use computers at all. But of course it's way too late for that. The horse has left the barn and has his own broadband connection with unlimited downloads.

The only solution is to teach children how to create ergonomic workstations and to use their computers wisely. That, combined with active and strict postural training. Of course it's also a good idea to limit their time in front of screens (including television). Inertia training shouldn't take up more than an hour or so a day, and it should be interspersed with stuff like riding bikes, playing ball, running around like a . . . well, like a kid.

PACKS AND BAGS

WE SHUDDER WHEN we see a tiny elementary school child
with a backpack nearly his size hanging heavily from his
shoulders, trudging toward school. Backpacks were originally intended to be easier on the back than other methods
of ferrying homework to and from school, but it hasn't
worked out that way. What has happened instead is that the
use of backpacks has contributed to the growing problem of
childhood back trouble.

Part of the problem is that kids often take too much home
with them, and there are books and pads and other things
they don't always need. There seems to be a universal belief
among children that every night you need to bring home a
pencil case filled with four hundred varieties of colored
pens as well as your own dictionary. Kids need to be
instructed by parents and teachers alike not to load themselves down with unnecessary gear.

And the backpacks themselves should fit and hang properly.
Weight is best carried close to the body, which means the
shoulder straps should be nice and snug so that the load lies
against the back at the top, not four inches away from it.
Otherwise, they have to walk leaning forward to counterbal-
ance the back-leaning load. It would also help if they used the
waist strap, but we don't think we've ever seen it happen.

There are more advanced backpacks with a support system
that loads most of the weight onto the hips and pelvis, but
they aren't regulation equipment in most schools. Not yet.

It would be better if weight were carried at the front of the
body, not the back. But once again, convention is not on our
side, and until there's more widespread recognition of the
damage done to our children's little bodies, we've probably
got Buckley's chance of forcing a change.

Backpacks slung over both shoulders are problematic

enough, but a lot of kids, especially as they get older, hang their bags from just one side. Probably because it looks cooler. This is a great way to acquire a serious case of scoliosis.

Instead of backpacks, some kids use sports bags for the everyday carrying of books, and don't even make the pretence of using both shoulders, so that all that weight pulls down on one side of their growing bodies. Once again, parents and teachers should be aware of the dangers, and incorporate ergonomic principles into school curricula and the planning of school environments. Perhaps you should even lobby your child's school to give them some formal tuition in good postural and ergonomic practices. Kids need to be taught from an early age how to look after their bodies so they can keep using them after they graduate. Otherwise we're going to have a massive crisis on our hands that is going to cost unimaginable amounts of money, jobs, and time. But worst of all, we could be creating a whole generation that will be largely disabled by chronic injuries and pain.

Homework

It's a common, almost adorable sight in any household with schoolchildren, especially adolescents: on the bed, your child sprawled on her tummy, propped up on elbows, her head bowed over a book. It's a sweet sight, but a disaster in the making. The static loading that occurs on the neck and upper back in that position is enormous. And that backward arch of the spine is all right for a stretch, but not if you hold it for a long time.

When your kids do homework, encourage them to do it in a position that won't injure their backs. And if you can get them off the bed, watch that they don't slump over their desk in a similar pose. Bribe them with food, favors, and even cash prizes, but get them into good postural habits now! They will thank you later and maybe even put you in a really nice nursing home when the time comes.

Pets

No, we're not talking about your pets' posture, which is usually great unless they have a disease or spend too much time at their laptop. We're talking about you and your back and how you can mess it up with bad pet-related habits.

Don't bend to put food or water in the bowl. Squat or kneel, bring the bowl up to the countertop and fill it there. And don't bend when you're playing with your pooch, kitty, or armadillo. Stand, run, walk, kneel, or lie, but don't bend.

If you have a dog that pulls or yanks hard on the leash, sign up for some behavioral training. Every tug pulls your spine off-center and can start a sequence in motion that could end in back pain.

Use it or lose it.

—Henry Ford

Afterword

e hope that was more helpful than it was overwhelming. We want to give you choices, not make you recede further into your cocoon of pain. Because for some people, that's what their back pain is—a little dark, a little cramped, but safe because it feels so familiar. They might have lived with their pain for so long that they can't imagine living without it. Like taxes, wars, and reruns, they've decided that it's an ugly aspect of life they'll learn to live with.

But in the huge majority of cases, you don't have to live with back pain. So get rid of that mind-set. Reject the victim mentality. And reject the notion that you're just getting older and this is the sort of thing that comes with the territory. It does only if you surrender. The choice is yours. The fact that you've read this book suggests you've already made the right choice.

Get out there and discover how to get rid of your bad back. There's a fantastic wealth of options from practitioners to exercises to nutrition and other ways to overcome your pain. It's just a matter of putting the right combination together.

Acknowledgments

*F*irst, I would like to thank my commissioning editors Jill Brown at ABC Books and Sue McCloskey at Marlowe & Company for their enthusiastic support, astute feedback, and aesthetic input. I'm also indebted to my sharp editors Geraldine Corridon and Jenny Mills, and Stuart Neal for jumping at the idea in the first place.

I'm also profoundly grateful to my agent, Deb Callaghan, for her unflagging support and guidance throughout my writing career.

I must also thank Kevin Cotter and Ruby Heery for vacuuming and hauling in groceries when my back was bad, and for their continuing encouragement of my literary endeavors.

I would also like to thank the many health-care practitioners who, over the years, helped me with my back troubles and fed me lots of material for this book. While they range across the full spectrum of therapies, each one passed on knowledge that helped me overcome my pain and I now pass this knowledge on to you. In particular, I'd like to thank chiropractors Leroy Perry, John Thie, and Jairo Rodriguez, osteopaths David Vivian Jones and Alison Masters, podiatrist Mandy MacDonald, general practitioner and acupuncturist Dr. Kit Lau, and Dr. Bernard Lake for his Feldenkrais training. Also the late Megan Williams, an inspired Pilates teacher whose voice I still hear when I exercise, telling me to keep breathing, and a very special debt of gratitude to remedial massage therapist Elsa Clut without whom this world would be a darker place.

Finally, I owe the most to my friend and osteopath, Peter Edwards, who contributed enormously to this book and who continues to help me solve my back problems when they sneak up. As both technical consultant and osteopath, he is dedicated, generous and imaginative, and I simply could not have written this book without him.

Index